DOCTOR UNDAUNTED
ANSWERING HEAD INJURY WITH HOPE

DON R. ROBINSON, MD

Copyright © 2020 Don R. Robinson, MD.

All rights reserved. No part of this book may be used or reproduced by any means, graphic, electronic, or mechanical, including photocopying, recording, taping or by any information storage retrieval system without the written permission of the author except in the case of brief quotations embodied in critical articles and reviews.

This book is a work of non-fiction. Unless otherwise noted, the author and the publisher make no explicit guarantees as to the accuracy of the information contained in this book and in some cases, names of people and places have been altered to protect their privacy.

WestBow Press books may be ordered through booksellers or by contacting:

WestBow Press
A Division of Thomas Nelson & Zondervan
1663 Liberty Drive
Bloomington, IN 47403
www.westbowpress.com
844-714-3454

Because of the dynamic nature of the Internet, any web addresses or links contained in this book may have changed since publication and may no longer be valid. The views expressed in this work are solely those of the author and do not necessarily reflect the views of the publisher, and the publisher hereby disclaims any responsibility for them.

Any people depicted in stock imagery provided by Getty Images are models, and such images are being used for illustrative purposes only.
Certain stock imagery © Getty Images.

All Scripture quotations, unless otherwise indicated, are taken from the Holy Bible, New International Version®, NIV®. Copyright ©1973, 1978, 1984, 2011 by Biblica, Inc.® Used by permission of Zondervan. All rights reserved worldwide. www.zondervan.com The "NIV" and "New International Version" are trademarks registered in the United States Patent and Trademark Office by Biblica, Inc.®

Tybee Island - Licensed Getty Images.
Robinson family announcement - *The Post-Searchlight*, Bainbridge, Georgia
Concussion - Concussion Vector Illustration Labeled Educational Post... Licensed Shutterstock image.
Sydney Lanier Bridge - Sydney Lanier Bridge jpg. Permission GCPCI project

Scripture quotations marked (NASB) taken from the New American Standard Bible® (NASB), Copyright © 1960, 1962, 1963, 1968, 1971, 1972, 1973, 1975, 1977, 1995 by The Lockman Foundation Used by permission. www.Lockman.org

ISBN: 978-1-6642-1034-9 (sc)
ISBN: 978-1-6642-1035-6 (hc)
ISBN: 978-1-6642-1033-2 (e)

Library of Congress Control Number: 2020921118

Print information available on the last page.

WestBow Press rev. date: 12/04/2020

DEDICATION

To the one who gave me her hand, her heart, and
her optimism. She has loved me to healing.
And to the Master of the Universe whose healing
hands provide hope in all struggles!

CONTENTS

Foreword ix
Preface xiii

Chapter 1   Introduction 1
Chapter 2   The Fall 5
Chapter 3   Running Day 9
Chapter 4   Training Years and Early Injuries 14
Chapter 5   Early Practice 25
Chapter 6   The Big One 31
Chapter 7   Symptom Profile 40
Chapter 8   First Clinical Steps 56
Chapter 9   Headaches 68
Chapter 10 Higher Level Evaluation and Care 77
Chapter 11 The Universal Therapy 85
Chapter 12 Lessons of the First Decade 94
Chapter 13 Honesty 102
Chapter 14 The Caregiver's Perspective,
            Introduction to Mary's Experience 108
Chapter 15 Mary's Experience 110
Chapter 16 Yesterdays 124
Chapter 17 Today 128
Chapter 18 Conclusion 132

Epilogue 137
About the Author 139
Glossary 141
Resources 143

FOREWORD

by *Chrisanne Gordon, M.D.,* Founder- Resurrecting Lives Foundation

> "The good physician treats the disease; the great physician treats the patient who has the disease."
> - *Sir William Osler, Father of Modern Medicine*

Dr. Don Robinson has gifted us all with his eloquent, very personal history of instant injury requiring prolonged recovery; of self-confidence replaced by self-doubt; of independence morphing into interdependence; of skillful surgery maintained by measured medical delivery. He invites us to join him on his journey of recovery from Traumatic Brain Injury, a journey we are very willing to take with him and his wife, Mary. In fact, we are pulling for him every page along the way, trusting that he will make it back to his former self. Changes came for the confident, over-achieving Ob-Gyn physician serving a small community in Georgia, after serving our nation in the United States Air Force.

We are with him! We are cheering for him! We are hopeful for his complete and utter recovery. We want this for him, not just because we all know someone who is still struggling with a brain injury or maybe we are struggling ourselves, but we want this for him and his family. His triumph over brain injury gives us HOPE for others, and perhaps hope for ourselves. We are willing to follow in his path.

"Physician, heal thyself" - Luke 4:23

Somehow, we believe that a physician, of all people, would be able to rebound from a simple slip in the mud, a slight bang to the brain. Certainly, he will blaze a trail for the rest of us, and, in fact, he does just that. The common factor in all brain injuries, however, is the change to the definition of "normal" and the rate of recovery, which is different for all of us.

Every year in the United States of America it is estimated that nearly four million people sustain Traumatic Brain Injuries (TBI). Thankfully, nearly 90% of these are diagnosed as "mild," as was Dr. Robinson's. That is, no gross abnormalities are discovered on routine testing such as a CT scan or MRI. There is no external sign, either, making these life-changing, invisible wounds so difficult to overcome. Indeed, nearly 750,000 young men and women from the conflicts in Iraq and Afghanistan, the most fit population in our nation, are struggling even today with issues of memory, processing, concentration, balance, and what Dr. Robinson aptly names, spatial insecurity. Often accompanying TBI, and, in fact, dependent on a brain injury, is that entity named Post Traumatic Stress Disorder, PTSD, which causes further distortion and disorientation, especially when challenged with hyperstimulation such as at sporting or entertainment events.

How does Dr. Robinson heal himself? He doesn't. He's smart enough to realize, almost at once, that he is off-balance, literally and figuratively. He is sustained by his Faith in God, the Higher Power, to regain his talents and continue his practice as healer. He is supported by the Love of his wife and family. Most importantly for Dr. Robinson, and for all patients with TBI, he is driven by Hope. It is the skillful intervening in his story of these virtues, Faith, Love, and Hope, that gives meaning and substance to this book, this labor of love. By his own example, he is teaching us how to recover.

One of my favorite phases, in what I consider a brilliant manuscript of memorable prose, is when he mentions that a neurologist, a physician trained to diagnose and treat TBI, told him to keep running. Now, Dr. Robinson ran marathons and half-marathons, and was, literally, dealing with significant cerebral fatigue at the time. He mentioned that she was probably speaking more in theory than in practice. It is sound advice and a caveat for any patient seeking assistance for brain health. What we learn in medical school and post-graduate training does not always translate to patient care. We are discovering that when you are "out of your brain" you are not "out of your mind." So, phrases like "press on" and resilience, mean nothing to a brain whose nerve networks are not firing.

One of the more important chapters reminds the reader of the need for validation, the need to know that you are not "out of your mind." As a physician, Dr. Robinson did not get this validation from his physicians very often. So, how much more difficult would it be for the non-physician, for the young veteran back from combat, or for the young woman beaten by domestic violence? In other words, if *he* wasn't validated, how can these patients expect to receive reassurance that they, too, have an injury that will improve with time and therapy? Here, Dr. Robinson is speaking to his profession: "Treat the patient who has this disease."

Dr. Robinson invites his readers to continue to *hope*. Although he was supported by a broad network of medical specialists and colleagues, as well as family and community, he realizes that the vast majority of those four million injured patients/year will not have this vast support system. In addition, access to medical care will be more limited for the vast majority due to finances or distance from care. Even now, there is a reluctance in major systems, such as the Veterans Administration Hospital and the NFL, to support the invisible wounds sustained on the battlefield or the playing field. We can and must do better to educate administrators of major health care systems, as well as the physicians they employ.

As a physician who, like Dr. Robinson, sustained and recovered from a traumatic brain injury, I salute him and his family, for his courage to come forward with this story, complete with the deficits he noted, the frustrations he experienced, and the *faith* that carried him to recovery. I recommend this book with highest regards. In the medical profession, it is rare to encounter such honest writing about shortcomings, and even rarer to see it reported with such eloquence and courage.

PREFACE

Thank you for picking up this book. I hope you will spend some time here. This book came about as I reflected on the lessons I learned through a time of uncertainty in my life. I suffered a head injury that significantly altered my experiences and relationships in 2004. This book you are holding tells about my injury and how I felt its impact. These pages are more than just documentation though. This is also the story of wounding and healing, frustration and fight, despair and devotion, and oh, so many other lessons! We will reflect on how the events of one day can impact your life for years to come. As you read, be sure to note that before I could really make progress in healing, I had to redefine the portrait of my self-image. My original portrait of self was shattered by the sequelae of head injury. My capabilities and tolerances were no longer the same as they had been in the years before. I had to learn what was different about the new me, what adjustments were needed to compensate and recover, and how my priorities would need to be reassessed.

This all occurred during a time that I served as a busy small-town doctor, answering emergency calls and delivering babies. This is the story of going from learning to survive the insult of injury to learning how to thrive as a new creation.

I hope to share with you lessons I learned on how to accept, adjust, and continue the fight. Additionally, there is a bigger picture here. My journey into healing also taught me lessons of loyalty, love, and grace!

If you, too, have suffered a roadblock on the avenue of life, you may see yourself in my journey and its challenges. If you know of someone who has literally been staggered by a head injury, I will hope that this story provides enlightenment and encouragement. If you are a caregiver, maybe this will help you to understand and to be understood. My wish is that the lessons I learned from my battle may tool others in their efforts to overcome!

CHAPTER 1

Introduction

"I learned that I was never alone, that there was Someone always very close by and, indeed, within me, giving me strength in times of weakness and desolation, light in times of darkness, joy in times of great sorrow and pain, and the will to struggle on when continuing seemed futile." (From My Struggle with Faith by Joseph F. Girzone)

I didn't remember her birthday.

<u>I didn't remember her birthday!</u>

I DIDN'T REMEMBER THE DATE UPON WHICH MY BEAUTIFUL BRIDE WAS BORN!!!

I was shook! But let me be sure to be correct here. I don't think that I had truly forgotten her birthdate. I had learned and relived her date of birth since we met in 1971 and through nearly thirty years of marriage at that point. I think the more accurate statement would be that I couldn't recall or bring forward her birthdate from my memory bank. There is a difference there, one we will explore along the path of this story.

Have you ever read a story that *started* with, "And they all lived happily ever after"? No? While we may wait to see if that phrase may be at the end, don't we all want to know how they got there, how the story played out? Isn't the story and life really about the journey? Well, this story of mine is from a long, incredible journey of pain and despair at war with determination, duty, and hope. If I had known what I would learn along the way, I might have been able to start the story with, "And we all lived happily ever after." Fate dealt me a hand with uncertain implications and unknown odds, and it was my place to play it out. I was initially in no mood to consider the happily-ever-after thing!

Mary, my wife, and I were visiting Savannah. It was all planned out. I was there to give a medical talk to residents and Ob/Gyn medical staff at Memorial Hospital. In fact, the subject of my talk was "Exercise During Pregnancy." I had previously given a similar talk in April, 2003, at a meeting of the American Medical Athletic Association, just prior to running the Boston Marathon. I was a big-time runner in those days. Understand, though, what I mean by "big-time runner." My dedication far exceeded my accomplishments! Still, it was a stress-reliever and something I really enjoyed. Being fit was a necessity if I expected any of my patients to listen to my preaching about health and weight control. The timing to give the talk was planned to coincide with the Tybee Island Marathon. You can guess the plan: lecture on Friday, enjoy the beach and food, and then run on Saturday! I also had been looking forward to introducing one of my son's friends, Matt Killough, to distance-running in a race setting. We were to run the half-marathon together. At least, those were *my* plans.

We will get to the details, but let's start here. This was Saturday. I had a fall the night before. As I remember it, Mary and I were just walking down the street that Saturday. I don't remember the conversation and I don't remember how the subject came up. But, there it was. I was struggling to think. What was her birthdate? I couldn't come up with that date. I had back pain and a headache, but what really concerned me was being lost in trying to find her birthdate among my brain files. That moment of loss, of confusion, of frustration, was when I realized something had started. I had no clue that day of the extent and impact that mild traumatic brain injury can cause, but I was beginning to be schooled! In fact, you will read later, as written by my wife's own hand, that my recollection of the setting here is not accurate. Yes, my reality was askew!

Actually, I had a background that set the stage for that day, but I had distanced myself from that history and thought it was no longer relevant. I thought that my prior injury history was all just old news. So, even though my challenge that Saturday wasn't really the start of all my difficulties, it was the moment I realized that there was something new and really different going on! My way of experiencing life was changing. More accurately, my ability to evaluate the world around me was vastly different and had changed dramatically. I am glad that I didn't fully comprehend the extent of that change, how it would develop, or what it would mean! What came before that day, and what came after that day, make up this story. It has all been a series of alterations that diverted my path in life in many ways. Little did I know the journey was on! As I look back over the last fifteen years, I am thankful for recovery, however slowly it may have progressed. I have learned so much along the way.

Why would I take the effort to write this down as a book? Am I bored? Am I self-possessed? Do I think I have all the answers? None of those suppositions are the case here. I will confess the truth to you, though. I recognize that there have been a few key times in my life when I just knew what I was supposed to do. This is one of those times. Going back, I knew I was supposed to be a doctor. I knew I was supposed to marry my wife. I knew I belonged in little ole Bainbridge, Georgia, a place I had never even seen before that directive became clear to me. While I may not have always recognized the Master's hand clearly at the time, I most certainly see where those convictions have led me. I give Him all the credit.

Now, I am convicted of the need to reveal my experience in this form. I feel the urge to share what I felt and what I learned through concussion, post-concussion syndrome, and vestibular dysfunction. I am choosing to reveal myself and outline my journey. There were many times along the way that I felt lonely. I wondered if there were others struggling like I was, if there were others that got strange looks from some doctors, if there were others that might be as "far out" as me. I want to let you know that the world of concussion and mild traumatic brain injury is *real,* and the effects are *real*. In some, symptoms resolve quickly. In others, such as myself, that is not the case. There is no good definition of what you may experience or how long it may last. There can be times when hope and despair may do battle within you. As you struggle, there may be times when you wonder: when will it get better, will it ever get better?

I have learned that there are other victims who are going through experiences that can be discouraging. I am reaching out to help those with similar challenges. I do not have answers for you as to what and when. What I do have is *hope*! What I can share is that I have continued to improve over the course of fifteen years. While you may not want to hear that it can take that long, what you need to concentrate on is that there is a continual reason for hope and optimism, day after day.

What I experienced and what I learned have worked out for the good. I want to share that discovery of joy with you. I have grown to realize that my story is not that unique, although in the early days that was unclear for me. Just maybe the time we spend together here will ease your concern. Maybe my lack of uniqueness is the point here. Maybe that just makes this story worth the telling.

Often, as we go through difficult times, it helps us to find how others have trod similar trails. While we may be at different signposts at any one time, as we look behind or see ahead, we can note well-worn paths. As we look forward, we can gather crumbs of hope, realizing that it is possible to successfully navigate the course ahead. Whatever challenge you may face, you are not on a journey that others have not experienced! There are indeed common paths. You just have to find your path among the many, the right path of positivity for you to follow.

Where will you turn? Some are tempted toward alcohol or drugs, to deep despair, or to defeatism. I don't have to tell you that those are not healthy alternatives.

Here, let me help you answer some questions:

"Can I go on?" Most definitely!

"Will it get better?" Most assuredly!

"Is there hope?" Most emphatically!

You must turn to those who love you, to those who support you, and to those who accept you! The heart of humanity, the strength of the Spirit, and the expertise of professionals will guide you. You are not alone!

CHAPTER 2

The Fall

"Everything can change at any moment, suddenly and forever." Paul Auster

The year was 2004, the month was February, and the setting was Tybee Island, Georgia. Mary and I had traveled to Tybee Island for a short chance at relaxation. At the time, I was in active medical practice in a small town in southwest Georgia. I needed a break. Being on call every second or third night as an obstetrician and gynecologist is a tiring, sleep-disturbing way of life. We headed to Tybee to give a medical talk, to enjoy the island, and to meet up with a friend for a running event. A little time off and a lot less stress for a few days seemed to be a *wonderful* plan. Why wouldn't that be *great*?

Well, the talk Friday morning went OK. (Doesn't the speaker always think that?) My hosts were gracious, and the audience was receptive. I always found it fun and exciting to share knowledge. Studying women runners has been very essential to making safe guidelines for active women. Many mothers-to-be are excited to be moms, but they plan to add that blessing to their already active lives and journeys. Often, women want to continue their training during pregnancy and renew their efforts, as soon as they can, postpartum. Along with the crib, they may order a runner's stroller. Researchers have worked to define the safe ways to accomplish these multiple goals. I had studied this and was always willing to discuss and explore.

Mary and I had an outing planned later that day, Friday night. I love seafood and I love restaurants that are rustic. Usually, I find that picnic tables, especially those with a hole cut in the middle for empty shells and well-picked bones, are a lot of fun. Those relaxed environs are often the home of true American seafood greatness! We selected such a place that night, hidden down dark roads on Tybee Island, an island just off the coast from Savannah. The restaurant scored high on the rustic meter! In fact, it was really a shelter with a roof, screen walls and door, and restrooms across the yard (or mud that night). The only way to be more primitive would be to add darkness and rain. Both of these realities presented themselves in abundance that night.

My son, Tal, had already left the nest to pursue his life, but we still had relationship with some of his friends. One of those friends was Matt. Matt was, and is, a great young guy. He is an adventuresome sort and was just getting into more serious running. He knew I had run several marathons. Months earlier, we began talking about running at the Tybee Island Marathon, doing the half-marathon together. I gave him some small amount of advice on training, and he took it from there. Our plan was to meet at that rustic seafood dining experience for a pre-race dinner. It wasn't a pasta meal, but it wasn't to be missed, either! Excellent seafood is a basic joy and right, after all. Wouldn't you agree? A relaxing, restful experience with scrumptious food. That was my plan. However, events didn't necessarily follow my plans. That is really when and where the injury happened. And the course of my life was altered.

As I reflect, I realize that we often fool ourselves with plans. God lets us realize, sometimes easily and sometimes hard, that our plans are just dreams, often without any actual foundation. We are not truly in charge of our own lives or our futures. We never know when our life path is about to take an unexpected turn. That turn may occur in an instant, or even a fraction of an instant. Just as a stream will find its way around a boulder dropped in its path, we have to find our way around circumstances that are totally unexpected and outside our thoughts of the possible. That unexpected event may be a shock, but it may also make for the adventure of your life!

I remember the restaurant on Tybee Island where we went for supper. To say it was rough is like saying a cactus is a little prickly. The structure may have been very primitive, but isn't it really all about the food? The seafood was fresh and well prepared with lots of fresh non-fried options. It was just the kind of place I really enjoy: no pretenses. Just let me sit there and I can move through shellfish and shrimp, casting shells out of the way to go for more.

We all drove down a secondary road to this out-of-the-way place in the pouring rain. I must admit that pulling up in that heavy rain wasn't very enticing. It was a constant rain, no hope in waiting for a break. Our stomachs were demanding their due. We had to get out into a slushy, muddy parking area. You probably have been in a similar place. It was time to cover the head and make for shelter. We all managed our trek without incidence, even if we ended up somewhat wet! The crowd was down due to the deluge. We strolled over to a place to sit. I for one was full of expectation! I was now in a place of comfort that made me reminisce about joys of meals past in similar environs. Now it could rain all it wanted. We were relaxing. Food was ordered and eagerly anticipated. After all, with a race planned, one must load up with carbohydrates! It was my athletic obligation. Maybe you will buy that excuse for my gluttony!

It was time to wash my hands and prepare for the meal. When you dive into steamed seafood, clean hands are a must. There was just one detail: it was still raining like the clouds were exploding and that restroom was still outside! Well, I made it OK getting to the facilities that were located across a walkway. After cleaning up though, I had to return to the dining room to eat, now didn't I? It seemed to be raining even harder, like I was not meant to eat. I knew that was not true! My friends, I could not let that frustration happen. I set out to use that running skill of mine to quickly make it down the wooden walkway and back into the building. There was a slope down from the bathroom facilities towards the main wooden path.

I remember that path. It was open with no handrails. It was made from wooden boards, probably one-by-sixes, placed crosswise down the ramp and then flattening out just above the ground. Before I knew it, my running, fast-moving feet were moving even faster. They slipped on the wet wood. My assumption of traction became an assurance of anything but! My feet and legs flew out in front of me, starting my shoulders spinning back over my butt. I hit my back and my head, *hard*! I know I hit my back because it hurt me for weeks. I know I hit my head because I found myself dazed and looking up into the rain falling into my face. Was I knocked out? Well, I am not sure if I lost consciousness or not. My front was wet enough to say that I may have lain there for a while. Looking back, under the circumstances, I don't think I could have been out for any length of time over a few minutes.

Well, what do you do? No other disoriented wet folks were out there with me. It was time to get myself up, even if that was a challenge. I must have been quite a sight going back to the table to join Mary and Matt. I was wet on the front, and I was wet and dirty on the back. Let's just say it was the kind of place where such might not be as noticeable as at some other "finer" eating establishments.

I knew my back was hurting Friday night, and I knew I was a little fuzzy, but I was able to eat and get back to the hotel. I know I did not make a further scene anywhere. The rest of that evening is really something I cannot remember. This could be due to loss of memory from the injury or just because I did not take the evening seriously enough to make permanent mental notes of the situation. Either way, the recollection is just not there within my grasp.

CHAPTER 3

Running Day

"It is not in the pursuit of happiness that we find fulfillment, it is in the happiness of pursuit." Denis Waitley

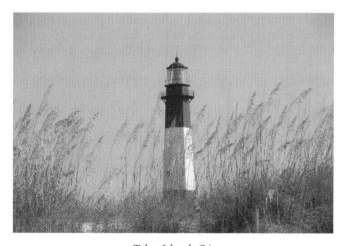

Tybee Island, GA

Tybee Island is a beautiful and historic place. It is one of the "Golden Isles" of Georgia. The most recognizable feature is the lighthouse, which has continued to be painted in its tradition of a white middle between a black top and black base, divided into thirds. I was expecting to view that lighthouse from all directions that morning. The lighthouse dates to 1736, bespeaking of the island's history in colonial days. I was counting on that lighthouse being my homing beacon the day of the run. This fact should not be overlooked! What I anticipated following that day was a man-made obelisk. My perspective of beacons to follow in the future was to be altered in many ways. One of those ways was to become more dependent on following beacons of spiritual guidance.

The native Americans pre-dated the arrival of Europeans by centuries. From pre-history through the Spanish and English colonial times, to the American Revolution and the Civil War, and even including World War II, the island has had an impactful place in the American story. The history surrounds you while the food comforts you. The seafood is primarily fresh, local catch and freshly prepared. During shrimping season, the shrimp boats are numerous and active. Because of the cut of the seabed, it can look as though a boat may be coming ashore in her quest. The standard of fried fish and shellfish are available, but so are other, perhaps more palatable, choices. And the beaches, well you just need to experience them. The Atlantic coast in this area is notable for fine sand, a very gentle slope down to the sea, and large expanses of beach open at low tide. The sea life is abundant, the bird life fills the skies, the marsh vistas are beautiful, and the seascapes are inspiring.

The marathon and half-marathon routes ran along a course that perimeters the island. It is an open and enjoyable course for the real beach-lover. The island is fairly flat, so no big hills are present. One does have to realize that it will probably be windy. It is an island beach, after all. Just remember, since the course is basically a big circle, if the wind is in your face on one side, it will have to be in your back on the other side, right? The marathon length is no longer available as a race at Tybee, but the half-marathon and other distances are still run annually. In fact, as of 2019, they offer five runs in one day, all adding up to 26.2 miles, the traditional marathon length. I was really looking forward to the experience of the race I was to run back in 2004. I wish I could have enjoyed the island more that fateful-day-plus-one.

I have shared with you how we were out to eat dinner the evening before the big run the next day. Remember, I slipped on a decline of a wet wooden walkway, while I was trying to run through the rain drops to stay dry. Instead, by trying to run, I ended up all wet! Maybe there is a lesson there about patience, a trait that I have been slow to really master!

Early the next morning, it was time to get up, get dressed, and head to the run. I had a routine down. Put on the singlet with the race number pinned in place, the running shorts, the correct socks and shoes, and the Runner's Lube to prevent chaffing. I had it all down pat by this time in my running career. I had completed eleven marathons, including three Boston Marathons. What a glorious experience that is to run into Boston from Hopkinton, on the trail of the greats! A beachy half-marathon in a relaxed setting should have been no big deal.

Well, it didn't turn out to be *no big deal*. It wasn't easy at all! My back was really hurting me. From the time I got up, through getting dressed, I was worried about how I would be able to run because of those back spasms. I did have a headache and I remember feeling a little confused. It is clear, in retrospect, that I didn't realize what was going on with my head. Hitting your head can create many varied and changing symptoms. Included in the injury spectrum I was experiencing initially was an inability to identify my limitations that day.

A lesson here is that you would think a doctor would know better. I did not, and you may not. It takes a while to assess the distinction between just *a bad day* and a real course-change in your perspectives. I was trying to ignore all I was feeling and power on through it. My head was perceiving my surroundings through funny filters, and strange input was confusing me. What I could not ignore, I was trying to minimalize and explain away. Persistence is just part of me, and probably part of you. Whatever happens, don't we try to always *normalize* and explain away? For me, that learned behavior of self-discipline and personal disregard was what all my medical training had prepared me to do. Sleepy, hungry, ill, whatever; you keep going. That, I believed, based on calling and commitment, was just a doctor's and a runner's lot in life.

Well, perseverance did not win the day. I only lasted two miles! Between the pain in my back and the fuzz in my head, I just had to stop for self-preservation. I remember being a little disoriented and concerned when I finally stopped running, wondering how I would get back to the starting line and my family. That was strange for me! I have always had a well-developed, keen built-in direction finder. I also was tooled with an adventuresome spirit, so that running in different directions was never intimidating. Boy, that disorientation was a sign to me then, being insecure only two miles from the start!

I never, before or since, failed to finish a race. It certainly was not the only time running affected my head. In fact, even though I tried to deny it initially, running always affected my head after that. I just tried to power through. I kept trying to overcome during my runs. I thought fitness had to be part of the answer to my feelings of disequilibrium. Much later, I was even advised by one of the sub-specialist neurologists that I should continue to exercise and run. I think she was one of those who knew in theory but not in practice. I took her advice to heart at the time and stamped my running pursuits: *Approved*.

I wanted to run. I enjoyed it. I always looked forward to taking my running shoes with me and investigating new towns and neighborhoods. At home, I had several paths and trails of different distances committed to memory. Being a runner was part of my self-image and part of my distraction/escape therapy. Those injuries at Tybee did not stop my running in the short term, but my joy of running was inalterably changed for the worse. Never again would I be able to run without being aware that my perception was being tainted. I found that as I took each step in my run, my head seemed to bounce just a little more than it should. From the standpoints of visualization, stability, and goals, this was making focusing exceedingly difficult. That false spatial alteration with each step, in turn, occasionally resulted in missteps and staggering as I ran. Missteps, or trips, yielded heavy compensatory steps to regain my balance and, thus, even more jolting and bouncing.

Despite these changes, in those months and years that followed the head impact, I was not ready to give up on running and I was not anywhere close to wanting to turn into a couch potato. Eventually, as my honest assessment of my condition could not be denied any longer, I did stop running for months. When I tried to begin again, with someone watching me for safety, I failed. That jaunting and pounding from running had just become too disturbing for my balance and perceptual stability.

As time has gone by, I have begun to be somewhat intimidated by running. I am concerned that I might have one of those falls that can occur unexpectedly by tripping or stepping awkwardly. I fear what will happen to my head with another hard impact. And I fear how long the change might last! After the struggles I have overcome, that thought is scary and limiting.

Matt went on to finish the half-marathon and I was very proud of his effort, especially since he did it all on his own. That may have been the last time he ran a flat course for a while. He lives in Colorado. I imagine him conquering new Rocky Mountain highs!

While Matt went on to conquer new heights, I was headed to a medical journey of many miles and years. My trail would also be uneven with multiple valleys and peaks. It wasn't until about three weeks after the fall that I started to really comprehend my injuries. We will get back to this point later.

SO, WHAT WAS IT REALLY LIKE? Early on, after the fall, I felt disoriented and confused. I really was more just resentful of this interference in my plans. Not having grasped the gravity of my injury and change, I was not scared or greatly disturbed. The day after the injury and the next days to come, I was really optimistic, anticipating I would be *normal* tomorrow.

CHAPTER 4

Training Years and Early Injuries

"They always say time changes things, but you actually have to change them yourself." Andy Warhol

I can't blame all my head problems on the fall at Tybee. If you are reading this because you have had some head injury yourself, you probably know that head injuries can be cumulative in effect. Our troops coming home from combat experiences are certainly aware of this, as are our modern-day gladiators: professional football players. The head is especially susceptible to repeat injury within the first few days or months. Football players' lives also document that repeated injuries over the years can have a cumulative impact, at least in some.

While my head injury history is insignificant in comparison to the experiences from combat or even from a stressful, head-banging career, my life may be more like what you or others have experienced. I hope that sharing what I went through, while attempting to stay highly active and committed, can be enlightening to others who are trying to keep going themselves. In fact, those of us who experience injury in everyday life may have much higher expectations of recovery, much weaker *excuses*, and much more difficult times getting support from others. With no *war story* or courageous sacrifice, we may receive the ole, "Get over it!" If only I could have!

As far as I know, I entered adulthood with no prior head injury of significance. When I was a small child, I played rough sometimes. I played tackle football in the neighborhood when my Mom could not see me. Who needs helmets anyway? I remember my brother assisting me in checking out a straw pile placed below a barn loft!

Childhood: everybody goes through it. Isn't it wonderful what protection and healing powers God has put into children? I could have been injured playing football, flying like Superman, wrestling with a dog bigger than I was, or who knows what. But I was not aware of any deficit. I did well in school. The only thing that held me back in the early years was my penmanship. Who'd have guessed that about a doctor-to-be, right? God gave me enough intellect to be in the running for educational opportunities and enough fight to compete with those who had even greater talents.

One issue of my childhood, that would have influence on my adult life, should be mentioned here, for further development later. As a child, I was one of those kids that suffered from *car sickness*. In my case, I am not sure that wasn't at least partially due to the times. I grew up in middle Georgia, in Macon. As we drove westward to Grandma's house, about ninety minutes away, we traveled in a car without air-conditioning. Both of my parents smoked, and they did so while we were traveling. Sitting in the back seat, in the wind, in the heat, and in the blow-by of smoke, may have raised my symptom level. I remember my father stopping the car. I would walk around, eating saltine crackers in hopes of stopping my apparent whining. The truth, though, is that children who suffer from motion sickness are at much higher risk of motion disorders as adults. That would fit my profile!

My first head injury that slowed me down was encountered on a night of call at Wilford Hall Air Force Medical Center in San Antonio, Texas. I was about twenty-four years old at that time and a senior medical student at the Medical College of Georgia. Because my medical school tuition and expenses were being paid by the Air Force, I had the opportunity to spend intervals on active-duty assignments.

Who wouldn't want to visit San Antonio, Texas? I was there several times during my military career. There is a lot of history there in Bexar County surrounding the Alamo and the Texans' great struggle for independence. There is also that wonderful river walk that snakes through town. To sit in the cool of the evening breeze watching the water flow is an all-time great experience. That, my friends, is a pleasant memory. Such interludes, between more challenging days of work, keep you going.

Allow me to digress here a moment and lay a foundation regarding the progression of training and education for a doctor-to-be. This will help clarify my circumstances and the point at which I was in my journey to becoming a fully-credentialed, specialty physician.

At Wilford Hall, I was serving a clerkship as a senior medical student, in my chosen specialty of Obstetrics and Gynecology. By the time of this clerkship, I had decided to pursue Ob/Gyn as my area of expertise. The required four-year residency training to become a specialist would begin the next year. The truth is that I was actually hoping to secure a residency spot at Wilford Hall. While circumstances with my family would change that path, in my clerkship I was very interested in working amongst the Ob/Gyn residents and attendings at that hospital. During my time there, I was motivated to do well as a physician-to-be. I wanted to learn and to impress, while setting the table for future options.

As a senior medical student (SMS), you already have two years of classroom education and one year of clinical experience under your belt. A SMS is more comfortable knowing his/her place in the hierarchy of education. That student has learned a bit about not looking so green to other staff, such as the nurses, as he/she develops clinical skills.

In most teaching institutions, such as those in Augusta, Georgia, where the Medical College of Georgia is located, and at Wilford Hall in San Antonio, Texas, there are always experienced professionals, supplemented by learning students. That goes from the one who draws your blood, to the one who gives you your medicine, to the one who offers you a surgical procedure. For the doctor ladder that I was climbing, the bottom rung is the junior medical student (JMS). You move up to SMS, intern, resident, fellow perhaps (if you desire to become a sub-specialist), and then become a fully-credentialed, attending physician.

Residents and attendings usually work full-time in their area of specialty. The JMS, SMS, and intern may all just be rotating through any given specialty field of service, for the sake of experience and breadth-of-understanding. Typical of doctors in training through those three years from JMS to intern, I served on the staffs of internal medicine, general surgery, orthopedics, pediatrics, anesthesiology, and neurology, amongst others. You may say, "I only want a *real* doctor." Please, have no fear of the one who is caring for you. There is oversight and supervision. Medical students and interns, those in their first three years of learning and increasing responsibility, are always subject to review and co-signing by more senior physicians. That should be reassuring to you. Many sets of eyes are involved in your care. What one may not perceive, another may see clearly. That may be a true benefit to the patient. However, it may also mean that you go through a whole posse of white coats at clinic visits or hospital stays. Physicians may only be licensed for independent practice after they complete the internship year. And they must meet testing parameters and other criteria. It is definitely a process, long and challenging. It certainly *should* be for those entrusted with helping to preserve your health and manage your needs in times of medical crisis.

Usually, after those first three years, doctors serve residency in their chosen specialty field, whether it be surgery, pediatrics, etc., or, in my case, obstetrics and gynecology. Back in those days, the USAF offered Ob/Gyn residencies at four of their medical centers. Wilford Hall was the only one I really was interested in pursuing. Thus, I arranged to serve there for the clerkship. Under the supervision of residents and attendings, I was learning and gaining experience. That meant I went to the clinic to see outpatients, I went to the emergency room (ER) to see urgent patients, and I saw patients in the hospital. While being part of the team of residents and attendings, I took care of laboring patients, I delivered babies, and I assisted in surgery.

Back then, an expected and essential part of any student, intern, or resident rotation was being on-call. That has changed some in recent years, because of the fear that medical errors may increase when *too many* hours have been worked. As I trained, taking call was just what you did, usually every third to fourth night.

We think of call as night duty, and it is. But it is more than that. You are on-call during the day prior to the night, as well. That means you go to surgery, clinic, or whatever your routine is. While there, you might also get *called* for any emergency or unplanned, unexpected patient need. After the usual workday ended, you stayed in the hospital and remained intimately available through the night. Your basic personal goals were simple: try to find time to eat supper and breakfast, try to find some sleep or rack time, and try to get a shower in the morning. Then you start another full workday. You worked that next day whether you slept or not, ate or not, showered or not. You just worked! That is just how it was, the accepted norm for a physician in training!

There is no doubt that this work schedule led to sleep deprivation, but it also led to a certain ability to manage under stress. It is a learned skill to be able to remain calm and think progressively when a medical crisis is occurring. The Boy Scout motto applies here: "Be Prepared." When you are needed, you must act decisively at times. This is true whatever the hour or your state of restful readiness. Developing that skill is essential, especially for those who go on to practice in locations where the medical providers are not stacked up the way they are in teaching hospitals.

Now back to my fateful event at Wilford Hall. I was on-call the night of my first notable head trauma. I was working with a resident, as always. We had all the patients settled down, the babies delivered, and the nurses' questions answered. After winding down a bit, we went to the call room to try and get some sleep. It was late, we were tired, and you just never knew what might be coming next. You did know you were working the next day. Sleep would definitely be helpful.

Shall I say the call room was sheik? Not exactly! You could call it a glorified closet! It did have two beds with clean sheets. They happened to be bunk beds. As was usual, the junior guy got the top bunk. The room was otherwise plain. Notable was one of those ubiquitous large, green government trash cans of the day. It was in the corner by the bed, looking uninvolved since there wasn't much of a way to generate trash in a *closet*.

Time was passing that night, and I guess I was pretty well asleep. The phone rang *loudly* in that small room. I was immediately at attention, programmed to respond! I was well-conditioned, if not well-oriented, perhaps! I reached for the phone; you always automatically reach for the phone! I rolled up on my side and stuck my paw out for the phone. I reached out as if there was a bedside table with a phone sitting on it within my grasp. Funny thing, though, I never have seen a bedside table for an upper bunk. There was not one there this time, either.

I was reacting out of conditioning, not thinking! Instead of my hand stopping on a solid table surface, it kept going *down* and I rolled right on out of that bunk and fell to the floor. *Bam* is right! I do not know what parts of my body took the impact of that fall, but I do know that my head hit right on the rim of that government-issued, steel trash can. The trash can held up just fine. You can be proud of your government contract in this case. That can was indestructible. Me, not so much!

I know I was dazed. I remember the resident's comments. He did answer the phone and respond to the nurse. He was hanging up the phone after saying something to the effect of, "Whatever you have out there, I have worse in here." He knelt over me, assessed me I guess, and helped me to get off the floor. I don't really know what happened after that! I am pretty sure I wasn't allowed to catch any more babies the rest of that night! The next day, I remember a headache but not much else. That was a long time ago now. Of course, I didn't know what was yet to come. When I said I wanted to make an impression during that Wilford Hall rotation, I did not have bouncing my head on a metal trash can in mind! That old saying… "Be careful what you ask for."

I completed that rotation, drove back to Georgia, and resumed my medical school education. I have no recollection of persistent symptoms after that injury. My lifestyle was such that balance challenges were at a minimum. I was pretty indolent in those days. I had married right before medical school and that wife of mine was trained to be a good cook. She had helped her Mom feed three brothers! Mary would fix large quantities of food for us to eat. After the first plate, then she would say, "That's not enough to save, *eat it*." Being the obedient husband that I was, I complied, of course.

Sitting primarily, for two years, studying my basic sciences at school meant I didn't burn a lot of calories. I wasn't into exercise at that time. And honestly, the volume of material I needed to study and learn was overwhelming. Medical school left little time for anything else. That extracurricular indolence pattern, avoiding exercise, even after I started my clinical rotations, was probably good for my head recovery. It makes sense to me that if you have an injury due to a sudden head movement or blow, it might help the injury to heal if you limit excessive jolting activities. I didn't really think about that then, but in retrospect it seems probable and plausible. Years later, after another injury, my progress, or lack thereof, when I kept running, seemed to verify this theory.

It wasn't really until a few years after medical school, when I came on active duty with the USAF, that I developed a fitness and exercise routine. That is partly because there were required standards, and it is partly because of my growing interest in fitness and weight control. Mary had always fed me more than enough for my needs. In fact, I think I was carrying at least one of her brothers' portions around my middle!

Life was busy and promising for the next few years. I finished medical school at the end of January 1980. I had worked through prescribed breaks at times, allowing me to complete the requirements ahead of schedule. I can't claim my life was all work! By the time we began residency, Mary was pregnant with our first child. Blessings were growing. I began my internship in March, and I was months into my training by the time of my medical school graduation ceremony in June of 1980. I went back to Augusta to take that walk across the stage. Even *that* was a story unto itself. I'll share that in a minute.

The only real reason I was there was for my mother. She had said numerous times that she wanted to be around for my graduation. Unfortunately, between the date I completed my requirements and the date I walked towards the dean to receive my diploma, she had lost her long battle with cancer. She certainly was there in my thoughts. One of the benefits I received by graduating early was that Mary and I were able to spend those last few months helping to look after and care for her. She lived in the town where I was doing my residency. We even had plans that she would move in with us. That never came to pass. She went from her apartment to the hospital and never came home again.

Still another aspect of my graduation stroll that made it rather unique was that the *walk* wasn't exactly a walk, it was more like a hop and a skip. I had injured my leg bone (tibia) playing softball on the Residency team, and I was in a cast. I left my crutches at the side of the stage, managed to get across, and then got back to my crutches. You can be sure that the leg injury as an intern made much more than just the graduation interesting! Crutches or not, I was rocking on through life and professional progression. Mary and I had moved to Macon, in central Georgia, for residency, and we were able to rent a nice house on a hilly lot. That hill and the steps figured prominently into my life when I later ended up having surgery on my hip and was blessed with yet another episode of crutches. Crutches and graceful moves just don't go together for me!

While work was hard and life was complex, my head was calm and quite functional. I had no residual or hint that my head was not 100 percent. Residency was a grueling journey through stress, sleep deprivation, maturity, acceptance of growing responsibilities, and confidence. That four years prepared me well for many professional challenges to come.

I completed my residency requirements on February 29, 1984. Yes, they made me work Leap Day! My next stop was with the United States Air Force. Two weeks after my last day in residency, I was on active duty and on my way to Wichita Falls, Texas, for an orientation, of sorts. My eventual duty station was chosen for me based on the needs of the Air Force. I remember I received a form to request my assignment preference. I listed four bases on the coast in the Southeast. Ha! When the Assignments Officer called me, he had a *better* idea. He sent me, as he said, "...to a place where I wouldn't have to keep my ice cream in the freezer." South Dakota, here we come!

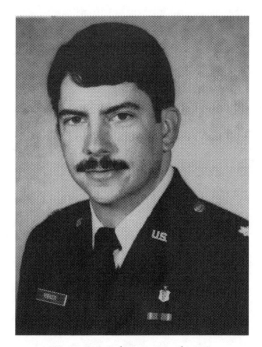

Major Don Robinson, Moody AFB

South Dakota is certainly a mixed bag. The landscapes are beautiful. The out-of-doors are inviting with numerous state and federal parks. Trout fishing was exciting. Mount Rushmore is inspiring. Keystone, the town located at Rushmore's base, is very entertaining. The problem was the limitations on the enjoyment calendar. Weather was frigid in winter, and the transition to and from summer was unstable and unpredictable. April and September weather could be surprising and downright dangerous at times. Blizzards and *for real* hailstorms are all too common. Sightseeing adventures were best carried out during June through August. Since my roots are in Georgia, relocating to South Dakota expanded my concept of reality.

I drove up from Wichita Falls, Texas, through a blizzard, becoming stranded along the way, in a place I do not think I have heard of since: Lusk, Wyoming. I became aware of why there are posts erected on either side of the road. I learned that in the aftermath of a blizzard the roadside and the road all looked the same dense white. You needed to stay between those posts! Following snowplows is also a talent I developed! Looking back, I really went through some threatening challenges on that trip. I guess at the time I was young and bullet-proof, or at least I thought so!

My wife and son flew up and joined me at the base. That first month was truly an adventure. The Northern plains were quite a change for my family and me. Yet another blizzard hit while we were temporarily housed in Visiting Officers' Quarters. That is when we learned that South-Georgia winter coats are not *really* winter coats *at all*. But that is another story for another day.

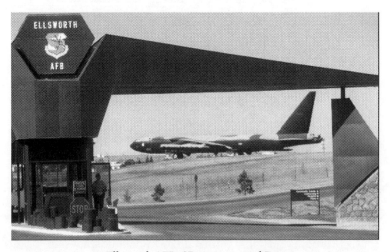

Ellsworth AFB, SD, entrance and B 52

The military base, while serving on active duty, was the site of my second exposure to head injury. And it was a more significant affair than my first encounter. It had been about six years now since the incident in Texas. I was on station at Ellsworth Air Force Base, near Rapid City, South Dakota. I was a full-fledged obstetrician and gynecologist. I had been working at the clinic and hospital there for quite a while before the injury. It was winter (wasn't it *always* winter?). I was walking into the hospital, across the packed ice, wearing my proper, leather-soled uniform shoes. Apparently, that is not a good idea! Next thing I know, I am doing a spin maneuver such as I would later accomplish/perfect on Tybee Island. This time, my feet went out to one side. There must be some principle here about feet sliding and the rapid acceleration of the upper torso. I can be the poster child! When I hit down, I hit on my shoulder. My head bounced, I gather, like a bobble-head! An airman saw me lying there and helped to get me up and into the hospital to be seen.

In a millisecond, I went from physician to patient. I was about thirty-one years of age at the time. I was in pretty good shape physically, but I'm sure I didn't look like much after a brain-bouncing fall. I needed the help which that airman provided. I was dazed and feeling lost. I needed support to walk straight.

I was seen by a primary care doctor in our clinic. He sent me home to rest for a few days. That was really the only option available then for treatment of a concussion. Our hospital did not have a CT scanner, so I did not get that or anything else done. Rest was the treatment then, and in many ways, it is still the best treatment!

Note of Interest: That day I was headed in early to perform some scheduled surgery on one of my patients. I did take time out to explain to the patient that it was in her best interest to postpone the surgery until the doctor (me) could see straight again. I don't know what I looked like, but she was easy to convince! Her convenience and planning aside, she must have seen true survival-value in putting off her surgery! There would be a better day for each of us.

SO, WHAT WAS IT REALLY LIKE? I have related to you the two falls. I had to clue you in. They are key to the story of the later injury. But those were just small blips of interest in the story of my life. As I discovered the fullness of life, I found adventure and success. My image of my capabilities inflated, and the image of my limitations deflated. Sure, there were long nights of studying or bedside clinical stress. Sure, there were rocky days in relationships. Certainly, there were discouraging days. Such things will always attempt to derail your journey. My self-confidence grew as I stayed on the tracks to my dreams. As my family grew, my success blossomed in sharing those joys! It was, and is, a great ride!

CHAPTER 5

Early Practice

"For I know the plans I have for you, declares the Lord, plans to prosper you and not to harm you, plans to give you hope and a future." Jeremiah 29:11

After my fall on the ice, it took a little while, but I resumed my routine. We worked hard in those days. During my assignment there, the Obstetrics and Gynecology Department at Ellsworth was staffed with two doctors and a midwife. We delivered *lots* of babies, primarily for the young airmen who were assigned to that base. At the time, Ellsworth was a base in the Strategic Air Command (SAC). The base was home to B-52s with nuclear payloads. Additionally, scattered all over western South Dakota, as I understand it, were Minutemen Missiles with their nuclear warheads. All that nuclear potential meant we had lots of security troops. Many young men, more than women then, who joined the Air Force were shuttled into security and some of those men and women ended up in South Dakota patrolling the perimeters. It seemed that one of the prime motivators for serving in the armed forces was to begin a family, or to support a family already begun. Those of us who delivered babies were honoring the commitment of these young people who were simultaneously trying to serve and protect their families and the country. It was a heavy commitment from them and for us.

I was on-call every other night and weekend for obstetrics and gynecology patients. I was also assigned to covering the emergency room a third weekend out of the month. That all added up to very little time off.

There were many nights and weekends when I never got home, snow or no snow. The worst experiences, I still remember, involved me being stuck at the hospital in active patient care. There was no cafeteria in the hospital. Food for the patients was prepared elsewhere and brought in for them. The hospital commander would not allow marooned staff, such as myself when I was actively caring for patients, to even buy food when it was brought in for the patients. Snack machines offered candy bars and chips, if that, as I remember. If my wife and child didn't brave the elements to bring me food, I was isolated, as if a desert island existed in the middle of that base.

When I wasn't working, we enjoyed our time in the wide-open spaces of western South Dakota. The Black Hills are exhilarating, and the Badlands are awe-inspiring. The morning after a snow was especially fresh and pure as you breathed deeply of the cleaned air. I must admit that natural high was somewhat offset by the need to shovel and re-shovel the driveway. It usually took about three days for the wind to calm and the sun to come out enough to crust over the snow and prevent it from continuing to blow and drift onto the concrete sidewalks and driveway. The base required me to keep those clean (around delivering babies) or I would be cited!

I could tell all kinds of stories about our time in the Northern plains, but my main task here is to let the reader know that I was young(er), robust, active, and highly productive. Despite the head trauma I experienced, I came back quickly and resumed my routine without any residual symptoms. I was two hits down, but I was sharp and effective. I had to be on top of my clinical game.

Did I say we were busy? My personal record there was seven babies in one night, from after dark to before sunshine! Anything we could not handle as young doctors in South Dakota had to be referred to Fitzsimmons Army Medical Center in Denver, Colorado. That is fine for a condition that needs to be slowly and carefully evaluated. Facilities in Denver, hours away even when an urgent flight could be arranged, were not much help when there was an emergency going on. Our small hospital had limited resources, no subspecialists, and no vascular or urologic surgeons.

I began to learn and mature in the art of early control of evolving medical problems. Preventing or managing medical conditions early to limit serious difficulties requires awareness, inquiry, suspicion, and the development of a sixth sense. There is a foresight that is required to help

DOCTOR UNDAUNTED

control a crisis before it really has a chance to snowball into something much worse. I had to be especially wary; *snowballs* are all too common in the Dakotas. Gynecology, but particularly obstetrics, is an area where acute changes and potential crisis are common. This experience in an isolated, but extremely busy, practice was essential in my later career in small-town South Georgia. I developed a term for this management principle that applied in South Dakota *and* in South Georgia. I called it practicing "frontier medicine." The primary medical motto has always been "Primum non nocere," interpreted as "First do no harm." That is universally accepted. My own personal motto that I adopted for small-hospital practice was this: "Be wary; avoid getting into trouble."

I finished my time in the service at Moody AFB in Valdosta, Georgia. Moody was in the Tactical Air Command (TAC). TAC was serious business, but there was more of an air of plenty. There was a somewhat more relaxed environment, with more ample resources, and, *Oh Yes*, a much warmer climate. No ice to deal with and, thus, a lessened risk for falls! I should have been a little safer, I was not sleeping in bunk beds anymore and people don't often slip on ice in South Georgia! I would eventually learn, however, that wet surfaces also have a challenging injurious potential!

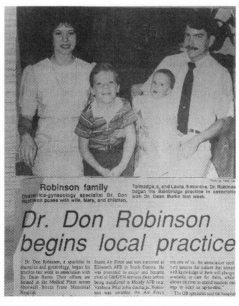

Dr. Robinson and family arrival announcement,
PostSearchlight newspaper, Bainbridge, GA

27

As my time in the USAF was coming to a close, I had arranged to visit several possible practice sites, primarily in Georgia and North Carolina. First on my schedule was Bainbridge. It turned out that visit was all I needed to see. I knew there were other good opportunities out there, but they weren't for me. The truth is that as I drove down the main street through town, Shotwell Street, I felt God's presence. I knew, without a doubt, that Bainbridge was where I was supposed to live and practice. I committed myself and my family without even really asking questions. It was just what I was supposed to do! I felt Bainbridge, Georgia, had been chosen for me, as the place to "hang out my shingle."

We discovered later, as we moved into town, that Bainbridge did have many assets. The Flint River runs right through town, making for boating and photographic opportunities. Bass fishing is king, with a mecca just downriver at Lake Seminole. The beach was two hours away and I replaced the North Carolina beaches of my childhood with the Gulf shores. For me, one who enjoyed birding and photography in my off-time, the setting was nearly ideal. There were bounteous opportunities for our kids to play ball, learn dance, etc. The biggest negative is a flying creature called a gnat. Gnats may only be less than an eighth of an inch in length, but they come in swarms and from all different directions at once. They have a propensity to head for moist surfaces on animals and humans (Don't think about that too much!). They live in abundance below the Fall Line of Georgia, which extends in a northeasterly direction from Columbus, through Macon, and up to Augusta. Below this line the soil is sandy, the residue of an ancient sea. Those gnats *love* it in Bainbridge. A hot summer day with gnats flying around your head, is not my idea of Nirvana. This is particularly true because they love to target my ears. I can't stand it! In fact, such days would provoke me to begin a conversation with God. Over the years, I would repeat many times, "God, You got me here. Please show me a sign as to *when I can leave!*"

With my Air Force obligation behind me, the doors to my new office opened on August 3, 1987. I had now reached my longed-for goal: the private practice of medicine in a small town. In Bainbridge, I joined a doctor, K. Dean Burke, MD, who began his residency in Macon about sixteen months after I did. As I went off to the Air Force, he completed his residency and then set up his office. At the time I was released from the

USAF, he was in need of an associate. And I was in need of a small-town practice not too far from an ocean.

By this time in my life and practice, I had so much behind me. I had completed medical school and all those exams and testing. I had completed my residency and survived the arduous process to become Board Certified. I had completed my pay-back obligation to Uncle Sam. At home, I had been blessed, through the tolerance of my wife, with a continually rewarding relationship, and we had been gifted with two healthy children. I had my first of several miniature schnauzers to round out the family. We had purchased our first house, nice but modest, on a quiet street in a good neighborhood. I had always envisioned raising my kids in such a friendly, close-knit community. We had settled down!

The "American Dream" was alive and well in my life and practice! A kid who started out with poor vision and scoliosis, who had two parents suffer and die from cancer, who got through high school and college in government-subsidized housing on Social Security Survivor Benefits, and who was fortunate enough to receive scholarships to fund college and medical school, had finally made it to his dream! After all those years and all that work, after building my skills and being blessed with a wonderful family, it was my time to pursue my medical practice and continue to serve others.

My goal was to build relationships, the way I had always hoped. I tried to practice patient-centered care. I learned much along the way about listening to patients. Doctors have notions about why patients get in their car and come to see them. If we are not careful, we medical professionals can zip right through the patient encounter thinking we have done our job. The patient, on the other hand, may be leaving the office wondering why it cost so much money for *that*? Having completed the prescribed steps of the visit, she may reflect on why she didn't get a chance to tell the doctor what she really needed! As a physician, one must pause and take time to recognize the goals patients have in mind, realizing that sometimes their goals can be very different from ours. Caring for patients, at its best, cannot be the prescribed time-limited, cookie-cutter approach that the managed care of today requires. To try and answer the patient's needs, one must listen, maybe listen some more, perceive, make eye contact, interpret, and serve. If the patient leaves the visit, having complied with our agenda, yet feeling that her needs were not allowed to be spoken or not taken seriously, then we have failed.

> SO, WHAT WAS IT REALLY LIKE? To be afforded such opportunity was *great*! To realize the talents and gifts I had been blessed with and to use them to serve others was *stupendous*! I felt comfortable in the Master's hands as I stretched my horizons to fulfill dreams. It was like being *thankful*. That is what it was like!

As I have stated, I began my private practice in 1987. I went from a partially full schedule that first week to more than I could easily handle by the end of that year. It was necessary, and turned out to be very rewarding, to develop a team with common interests in supporting our patients. A team of caring individuals, who may communicate in different styles and with different personalities, can really assist in facilitating patient care. Often, a clue that the staff uncovered, while getting the patient back for me to see, was passed on, helping me to identify the patient's real needs or reasons for coming. We had the luxury of loyal and long-term staff to serve patients from the first phone call, right through the visit. It was such a rewarding, if very tiring, small-town practice. Through ups and downs, business dealings, and patient challenges, the years were chugging by and my kids were growing up. Small-town life, where just about everybody recognized me, was full of rewards. As the saying goes, though, "The only constant is change." Just cruising along, day to day, you do not expect it. But watch out … change is lurking. And then - A BIG CHANGE HIT ME HARD!

CHAPTER 6

The Big One

"There are moments which mark your life. Moments when you realize nothing will ever be the same and time is divided into two parts: before this, and after this." John Hobbs "Fallen" **ILOVEMYLSI.com**

My third head injury, the one with the lasting results, occurred seventeen years into my career in Bainbridge. So much changed as a result of that injury. Let's go back to that time.

Three weeks after my third fall, I finally broke down and went to see an orthopedist friend of mine, Dr. Donald Dewey. His practice at the time was in Tallahassee, Florida, but he came to Bainbridge in rotation to see patients and perform surgery. We hung out in the same operating room at times and got to know each other to some extent. Also, he had helped me through several "overuse" injuries during my years of running, affording us the opportunity to build understanding. He had seen me tough it out through injuries before. But that day I was beaten; I was sitting on that exam table waiting for him to help me with my back. My lower-left back had been really hurting me ever since the fall, and it was not meeting my timetable for improvement (Have I told you I am not very patient?).

Dr. Dewey never really got around to checking my back. What I remember is that he was facing me while I sat on the table. He was standing directly in front of me. He never really stopped looking in my eyes. I remember that day was a bad day for my head symptoms. My "spatial insecurity" was acute. What he said startled me! He said, "Your back is not the problem, it will be fine. It is your head that I am worried about." Surprising to me, he didn't offer to do a thing for my back. He did facilitate my getting help for my head. He got a neurologist on the phone, and I was in the neurologist's office shortly thereafter.

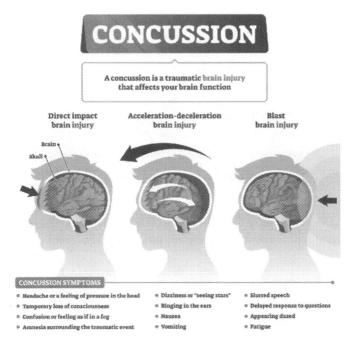

Concussion diagram.

Dr. Dewey said my eyes looked "funny" and I was having obvious nystagmus. For those of you who don't recognize the term "nystagmus," it refers to uncontrollable, rapid eye movements. This can be caused by many conditions; in my case it was the head trauma. In nystagmus, the eyes can move in more than one pattern. The most commonly seen manifestation, and the one I was exhibiting, is noted when vision is directed to the side. The eyes bounce back from the side to mid-plane and back to the side for several bounces. Let me restate that for understanding. You look to the side quickly. You are not aware of it, but someone looking at your eyes will see both your eyeballs bounce several times. The bounce is usually from the side back toward the middle, repeated for a few beats.

The more quickly the eyes are voluntarily turned to the side, the more involuntary bounces one may experience. This was three weeks after my accident. And apparently, I was doing some substantial "super ball" bouncing.

Many people incorrectly believe that whatever they experience right after concussion is the extent of what they will be dealing with. This is just not the case. With mild head trauma, it can take weeks for the full impact to manifest itself. According to a paper by Brandt in 1999, "The late onset of the symptomatology can be explained by the slow degeneration that sets in after concussion." I was seeing Dr. Dewey at a prime time for dysfunction!

If you have lived in the world of concussion, you may or may not understand my symptom terms. Those who have suffered like me, and have had such strange effects, can find it almost impossible to explain to others what they are experiencing. Communication with health care workers can be especially problematic. There are many professionals whom we may seek out for help, who know something in theory, but may be limited in their understanding of the practical reality! Family support may be a challenge as well. My wife tells me that there were times when she could not really understand what I was trying to explain. She has never had such an injury and has never personally experienced such symptoms. She could not feel what I was feeling or experience what I was experiencing. Her world did not contain a sphere of understanding for all of my head symptoms. However, she never doubted that for me, it was a very real alteration that I was trying to work through. As well, what she could see in me, she knew was real. Many times, she witnessed a vacant look in my eyes. That was certainly different from what she had witnessed in years past and different from what she expected. It was concerning to her. She was worried about me. And she was worried because she was uncertain about how our future might have changed.

She could see me cease movement and just be still at times. That was also very different for me. I was behaving in ways that she had never previously witnessed. She could note me being quiet. She might also see me standing with my back in a corner or holding on to a counter for stability. She could see my struggle. She could always tell when I was "spinning," as she would refer to it. That is probably a reasonable analogy, in that spinning tops do run out of spin and do eventually stop turning. I would eventually stop "spinning," as well, and be OK, but it would take variable lengths of time.

I remember that at one step along the journey, I developed my own terms for some of my symptoms. One of these symptom complexes I called "spatial insecurity." It seemed as though all I experienced from the environment was being inputted in different and, sometimes, strange ways. In fact, the new me was receiving excess input from my surroundings. I was really having a hard time focusing and staying on point, as the phrase goes. I was struggling with the reality of how my world had changed. My sensors were all turned open to the max, being overwhelmed, while being deficient in automatically filtering out background data of no real interest or importance. That is illustrated in the following story of another trip I took.

I thought this strangeness would just go away at any moment. Not understanding what was going on led me to conclusions that just didn't come to be. One of those false conclusions, based on a status quo that no longer existed, was that driving down the highway was easy and no big deal. Between my journey to Tybee Island, and seeing the neurologist for the first time, I had a trip to make. It was an obligation I had committed to before I ever went to Tybee. I saw no reason to not live up to that commitment. In my mind, I kept expecting tomorrow to be "normal." In fact, with this trip I had planned, I needed to travel back in an easterly direction within the state of Georgia again, this time to Brunswick. Tybee Island is near Savannah at the northern end of Georgia's coast. Brunswick is near the southern end of that same coastline. Each of these is about a five-hour drive from my home. I was headed to Brunswick for a medical meeting, driving by myself.

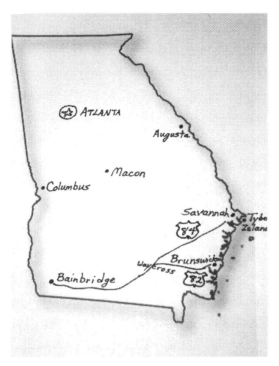

GA map detail.

You know, sometimes I say reality can hit you like being slapped with a wet mackerel! That trip to Brunswick was the wet mackerel, for *sure*, for *real*! I had been trying to carry on my work duties between the two cross-state trips. I had been doing relatively well, even if struggling. I am sure I was confused as to what was happening. I really had no clue as to the depth or extent of my challenge. Still, I expected all this would just be gone tomorrow. It turned out to be so many tomorrows! One thing I didn't appreciate then, and only really understood from reflection, is that many of my changes didn't start right away. Many of these symptoms developed over the course of weeks after my concussion. And some of those symptoms that *did* develop early on got more challenging with time. It makes it hard to target or comprehend the extent of your problem when it keeps evolving. In fact, what you conceive as a response to a need may require adjustment from week to week.

How can I dysfunction? Let me count the ways:

As I drove down the road, some things along the side of the road seemed to appear different from what they actually were. Bizarre was the new me! Just driving down the road, on a beautiful day, minding my own business, and voila, suddenly I see someone standing right at the edge of the road. I didn't note him as I approached, only as I went right past! It wasn't like he was jumping out in the road, but it still shook me. He who *wasn't* there, suddenly *was* there. How did I miss seeing him as I drove up, scanning the highway in front of me? In reality (as I discovered by looking in my rearview mirror) there was no man at all! What I suddenly interpreted as a man wearing blue and red was actually a mailbox on a post! That occurred more than once along that highway, misinterpreting a mailbox here or there, thinking each was a person, as I caught them in my peripheral vision. Each time, it was scary because it gave me the shocking impression that I may have just missed hitting someone along the road, someone I had not seen ahead of me as I was approaching. I knew better once I searched the rear-view mirror, and no one was there. But that did not settle my confusion. Hint here: I would suggest you gain the trust of your family or medical provider before you mention a symptom like this. The time I mentioned it to a sub-specialist, I got one of those you-must-not-be-right looks!

I remember driving down that long highway on a trip that was suddenly getting longer because of my confusion. Across South Georgia, there are many miles and wide expanses as you pass through tree plantations and mainly small towns. People, cars, and homes can be few and far between. What would it have been like if I had been driving in a congested municipal area? Ugly!

As the evening began to darken, mailboxes, etc., became less obvious and less intrusive. However, there was now something new to deal with. I had to focus straight ahead. When my glance wandered to the side of the road, the darkness made it appear almost as if I was riding on an elevated roadway. My perception was that the roadside just off the highway had a much steeper grade down away from the roadbed than what I had been seeing in the light of day. I *knew* that road. And I *knew* better. But my brain was being too creative, shall we say.

How can I explain this? During the day, my brain was failing to adequately screen out superfluous information, and that led to false assessments. At night, my brain was doing the opposite. It was filling in a new data set to supplement the lack of input from my surrounds. Instead of accepting darkness, my brain was being creative! Is that bizarre or what? As was once popular to say, I was now experiencing a "paradigm shift." Reality was no longer all it had been cracked up to be!

Motion was another issue that would cause me great challenges. One of the strangest things I experienced involved stopping at traffic lights. As long as I was driving fairly constantly, I could get by. But when I stopped, *oh boy*! Approaching the light, just as I had done when my life was more normal, I slowed down, stopped at the line, and watched for the green light. That is our programming and that is what it was supposed to be like. This time though, as I looked at the road ahead of me, it kept moving! I found myself pushing harder on the brakes, even though my truck had already stopped and was still. I could verify I was stopped by looking out the side window at stationary objects. Despite knowing that I was not moving, I was still seeing the road continue to move forward ahead of me. I had gone from seeing the normal of the road pass by to my rear, to the very abnormal of now seeing it run ahead of me. Shall I say that is a bit disconcerting?! Quite an understatement! What planet was I now inhabiting?

I knew, and I still know, that It had to be somewhere *in my brain* that the road image was still moving. Now that will unsettle you! I would just have to start the truck moving forward so that I could catch up with where my head had already led. I really did not want to stop anymore! Those were some lonely miles as the shoulders and the road played tricks on me! Yep, something definitely was malfunctioning. It was a new "real." It wasn't what I planned, it wasn't what I wanted, but somehow, it was definitely a new "real" and I had to overcome!

As a child, I suffered from car sickness. I have heard from multiple sources that those of us who have experienced such are more sensitive to motion disorders as adults. In fact, this is related by the VEDA group at www.vestibular.org. All of a sudden on that trip, I was a believer! I remember that same queasy, uncomfortable feeling of trying to adjust to movement, real and/or perceived. I had it as a kid and now I had it as an adult, but this time it had brought along its friend: perceptual distortion. By the time I went over the Sydney Lanier Bridge at the outskirts of

Brunswick, I was a confused and disoriented wreck of sorts. I was trying my best to be the tough guy who overcomes, but I *wasn't* overcoming. I was losing! For the one time in my life, I had a full-blown panic attack trying to get over that bridge. It is tall (did I say *tall*); one of those suspension bridges, and I am sure it is an engineering masterpiece. I have never really liked heights so much. And now, I did not like that bridge at all! With my newfound perceptual challenge of seeing the sides falling away, I was in a totally desperate land of insecurity. I was set up for a new, unwanted greeting from that bridge. I did manage to get to the other side, thank Heaven! I had to stop. I wanted to get out and kiss the ground!!! I made it to my hotel and checked in. No longer was I the man that I thought I was when I left Bainbridge. I was unsure of who I was, the realm I was living in, and what had happened to my capabilities. The battle was *on* in full force. I was a basket of insecurity, suddenly fearful, looking within myself for answers. I did not turn to my spiritual side as I should have in such a crisis.

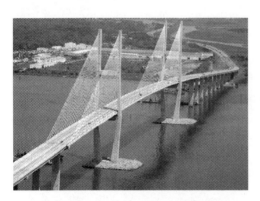

Sydney Lanier Bridge, Brunswick, GA

How about an aside here? My YouVersion scripture for the day, the day I am recording this, just came up: "No temptation has seized you except what is common to man. And God is faithful; he will not let you be tempted beyond what you can bear. But when you are tempted, he will also provide a way out so that you can stand up under it." (I Cor. 10:13) My temptation that I succumbed to that day was self-will, trying to handle it all myself, as if I could find all the solutions, short of God. Boy, was that a concept sure to fail!

I spent my few days in Brunswick and then returned home. I took a different highway home and did not confront that bridge for a few more years. Let's just say it made an impression on me. That bridge was a climax to a scary day. My new world was revealed in ways that had rocked me. The trip back home was no different, except that I was not totally surprised by these strange happenings. I also traveled all during the day so that I only had to manage the daytime-set of weird.

SO, WHAT WAS IT REALLY LIKE? It was terrifying. It was heartbreaking. It was like walking home for miles with a basket of eggs, only to drop and break them on the threshold. The most outstanding feature really was not even the troublesome symptoms. It was the uncertainty and insecurity I was left with. Thoughts of "where do I go from here?" had some disturbing options! I didn't really want to consider the possibilities.

CHAPTER 7
Symptom Profile

"Ships don't sink because of the water around them; ships sink because of the water that gets in them. Don't let what's happening around you get inside you and weigh you down." Unknown

There was a time when I was reeling from what was happening. I was waiting to see what the next bizarre act of my brain would be! It was almost as if my brain wanted to create its own variety show, with different acts to keep me entertained. Well, I didn't find it very entertaining. I found it distracting, and that was not a good thing!

I continued to do my duty, to see patients, and to take call. The real difference was that I began to feel insecure when I was called upon to provide more complicated care. My knowledge and judgment base were not impacted, but sudden movements could start me spinning! One thing a woman in labor is prone to is sudden movement. At times, I was literally holding on for stability, reaching out for a bedrail, a wall, or a knee brace. I also figuratively reached out to the nurses I worked with, as well as to my partner, to make sure that I had adequate assistance and back-up. I had too much God-given opportunity to quit, but I also had to make sure I was under control and safe in administering care!

Let me try my best to describe the feeling of "spinning." Spinning would occur with an unexpected or uncontrolled movement. It could happen with a sneeze, an adjustment to traffic, a door closing in my direction, or someone approaching closely in an unexpected way. I told you about those bothersome gnats. They love eyes, mouths, and ears. Ears are the worst! There was more than once that I would react to a gnat at my ear by slapping the side of my head reflexively. When you have a spinning disorder, slapping yourself is definitely *not* in your best interest!

Whatever the input, it would cause my brain to zone out for seconds to minutes. It really involved shutting down reactions. Instead of turning my head in greeting to that person who approached unexpectedly, my perceptions would freeze just like a video being paused. My head would tell me not to move so that my input would stabilize. The tilt-a-whirl effect had to balance out in order for me to go on. I rarely had true vertigo, as in seeing everything around me moving. I just had shut-down and an inability to be, shall we say, my usual witty and charming!

Did you know that sneezing could be dangerous? Neither did I, but I found out it was for me. We all yawn, cough, sneeze, etc. These functions are a part of everyday life and bodily function. Any of these can be more extreme at times. Certainly, coughing and sneezing increase with upper respiratory infections. They may also increase during allergy season. In South Georgia, we grow peanuts, corn, and cotton in abundance. That is because we have a long growing season. We also have two prime flowering seasons: the spring and the fall. As you have experienced, there are sneezes and then there are *sneezes*! Let me tell you, one of those big *sneezes* can take me out of the game. I can start spinning to such a degree, it feels like I have gotten a fresh concussion. It may take hours or days to resolve the aberrant crescendo of feelings.

Riding in a car as a passenger has its own set of challenges. When you are the driver, you know when you are going to turn, slow down, or make an evasive maneuver. The driver can anticipate, brace, and prepare for the forces coming. As a rider, you cannot anticipate, you can only react. For the subtle forces in driving, such as changing lanes or pulling up to a stop light, this may not be an issue. If, however, the driver has to brake hard to avoid a car pulling into the lane without warning, the unexpected force can literally be disturbing. I never figured out a way to do better in dealing with those sudden changes.

To this point, I have described the world of the weird and the bizarre that I experienced while driving to Brunswick on that first road trip after my injury. In the last paragraph, I described how tough it can be just being a passenger in the car. So far, you might surmise that cars were not my friends! Well, since the mission of vehicles is motion, and since motion had become my nemesis, that is a predictable challenger. I found, though, that there can even be hazards when the car is cruising at a constant speed on a smooth road. Remember, I was also susceptible to visual stressors. That was evident in how I reacted when a person suddenly popped around a corner into my view. Startling, up-close, visual impositions would stir my spinner! In a different way, there was even another visual phenom that got my attention for the worse.

In the area in which we live, as we drive down the road, we often go through forests. In fact, there are many square miles of national forests and corporate-owned forests, in South Georgia and North Florida. You may have noticed that many of these areas are what are called pine plantations. These particular lots have been planted with slash pines, or some similar variety, to produce the fast-growing pines that are most profitable in the manufacture of paper products.

When these pines are planted, they are planted in rows like other crops. What all this means is that when you add the sun rising or setting behind these tree rows on the side of the highway, you get a strobe effect washing over the car that can last for miles. Strobe lights are known to be hard to handle. In fact, strobe lights can be used to provoke aberrant waves when an EEG is being performed. Have you ever tried to move one of the car visors in order to block that sun strobe? You may be able to block your actual view of the sun, but the car will most likely still be bathed in intermittent, pulsating, bright light and dark shadows: off and on, off and on. That can confuse your sensor, and it did mine. It gave my mind extra data to deal with and limited my ability to handle other thinking. Result: Yet another reason to move over to the passenger seat! And, unfortunately, another reason to stay home.

Oh, and I used that term "spatial insecurity." You could use other terms, such as disorientation to your surroundings, but spatial insecurity just fit. As we go through our day, our brains are constantly filtering and interpreting what our eyes are seeing. For example, you may see a bush. All of the leaves on your side of the bush are there, and you could count them if you so desired. While they are in your field of view, they are not what you are looking at, so you do not really notice them. Your brain, when it is functioning normally, filters data and makes assessments, subject to override, without you having to make a conscious thought or directive. Your brain knows you are not here to count the leaves. You have other things on your mind and all you need to perceive is that it is a bush to avoid walking into. You see, perceive, and move on in microseconds. Your brain assesses relative value, based on your needs at the time, and generates a thought to the effect of, "Forget the bush; watch out for the snake and stay on the path," kind of thing. As my friend, Dr. Chrisanne Gordon, phrases it, our brains let in more input because our tool to fine-tune data is damaged. She relates that she believes that letting in more data is a protective response to the loss of discretion. My calling it "spatial insecurity" is based on the observations that it is difficult to function when you can delegate so little to background to be taken for granted.

In the example above, you are really ramping up the level of data complexity when the bush is not a single data-point but, instead, is a set of 100 or 1,000-plus data-points requiring continued analysis. When your senses are not comfortable assigning items to the background, such as ignoring that bush, ignoring that wall, ignoring that door, ignoring that counter, or being content with that mailbox at the side of the road, your mind becomes inundated with data. That data is missing the discretion of prioritization. Your mind, or computer control, gets bogged down in data-overload mode and has difficulty with processing it all. Sometimes the mass inputs can even force a shut-down. That is why I stopped driving in traffic! A driver who is prone to reacting with blank stares in traffic is not healthy or acceptable.

As I will discuss later, I was trained never to use the term "dizzy." I was told it was too non-specific and subject to multiple definitions. It could mean something different to each of the people that complain of suffering from it. In a way, all of the terms I use are in need of definition. My symptoms and your symptoms may be close to the same, and yet, we may use totally different terminology to discuss them. That is why I am trying to include more explanation when I use terms for my issues. I read in a medical article, "Vestibular Disorders Following Different Types of Head and Neck Trauma" by Kolev and Sergeeva, published in the journal, *Functional Neurology*, that after mild head trauma, "dizziness" can last at least two years in up to 18% of those affected. Count me part of the 18 percent, however you define dizziness. How about you?

My life was quickly being modified. My office assistant knew that if I moved the wrong way or at the wrong speed, she would just have to give me time. My partner, Dr. Dean Burke, may not have understood what I was experiencing, but he was willing to be with me in the operating room when I needed a safety net. The other nurses in the office may have thought I was strange anyway. They never really questioned my going to sit in a corner for a few minutes. And oh, that wife of mine. She knew that when I got home, I was done. I hit the chair; that was all I could do. Eat dinner or not, it did not matter. I remained still; I did not want to move. I wanted to stay frozen in the chair, and sleep would frequently overtake me. My head was demanding many more hours of rest.

I mentioned the term "motion disorder" earlier. You may find more information under the term "balance disorder." This condition represents a whole spectrum of symptoms and difficulties. I well remember being "car sick" as a child. I remember my mother trying to find solutions. We tried stopping, saltine crackers, who knows what. The car sickness was just part of my world. It was obvious that my older brother did not suffer the same ill feeling. Yet, fortunately for me, that sickness while riding improved for me with age. As an adult, I had no symptoms while driving or riding in a car, prior to my last fall. I assumed that my motion-sickness problem was just better, and it would always be that way. I thought I had outgrown it. HA!

I am sure I must have always had the motion-sickness tendency, even though I had adapted by somehow keeping it below the surface of my consciousness. I never got to the point where turning in a circle was not an issue. When we would go to county fairs or adventure parks, I could ride roller coasters with the same fear/joy equation as others. However, I stayed off anything that went around in circles. Picture the teacup rides. Not for me! That would make me miserable, to the point of vomiting. Picture a doctor who happens to be green in color! That could be me! It is not good advertising for a doctor in a small town to appear in public, staggering, looking "drunk as a skunk."

I had no issues flying in planes or helicopters in the USAF. It was just that around-and-around thing that would do me in. I could avoid the fair. I could avoid the teacups, the Scrambler, and the other around-and-around rides. That is as easy as not stepping into a mudhole to prevent getting your foot wet. The trouble was that here and now I was experiencing the effects without ever getting on the ride. It was not a matter of avoiding stepping into it, it was a matter of trying to step out of it. I could not avoid the sick feeling when it was internally generated, and my brain wasn't playing according to the usual rules. That is where I was at, after the last fall. Those were some miserable days.

I do not know if anyone else out there has experienced this symptom as I have. I wonder. When I was fresh in the morning, I could easily drive the two miles to work at my office in Bainbridge. No real problem. My mind would be busy with where I needed to go first. Did I need to make rounds, check on x-rays, assess patients in Labor and Delivery, see a consult, or go to surgery? I fooled myself into thinking I was "large and in charge." But by the end of the day, however, I was doing well to just get home. It was as if I had given it all at the office! By between 5:00 and 6:00 p.m., there was nothing left. My tank was empty; the gas was gone! I would concentrate with whatever brain power I still had, in order to drive safely home.

I would pull into the carport and just sit still in my truck, grasping the steering wheel until the world around me stabilized. There was discomfort in the pit of my stomach. My family might come out to help me in, or they might just give me a few minutes. Actually, it was better for me just to sit still and recover. If someone came out to help, I would feel guilty and get out of the truck before I was really ready. Given my own time, I would settle down enough to pick up my stuff and walk into the house. My energy was gone, my stability was shot, my ability to concentrate was kaput, and my energy to interact was absent. Without an adrenaline rush caused by an emergency, the only thing I could really do was sit and vegetate.

For the most part, I slept well during this time. I would struggle with restlessness during the night occasionally, but not most nights. I was on-call about every third night, and that certainly contributed to wearing me down. When I was needed at the hospital, my wife was always alert as to whether I needed her to drive me in or not. Most of the time I felt safe to handle driving by myself, but she was there; always there!

Brain exhaustion was real and dominating for me. Before my injury, I used to always leave the office at lunch to go home or to a meeting of some sort. Now I needed to utilize that time to sleep. Right there in the bright, fluorescent lights of my office, I would put my feet up, rock my chair back, and take a nap (or at least rest with my eyes closed). The constant light did not seem to bother me. In fact, leaving the light on saved me a trip to get up to turn off the switch. Occasionally my nurse would come by and switch them off.

I usually had an apple and either some crackers or a snack bar for a lunch effort. I set my alarm to rouse myself just before patients started back. I did other things to conserve. Before my injury, I would always start my day at the hospital to get a feel for how our patients were doing, whether I was on-call or not. After the injury, I adjusted to phoning on the way in and only showing up if I was needed. After a tiring day, before I went home in the evening, I might make phone rounds instead of going to the hospital, if I was told all was quiet. That would save me from driving over there with additional starts and stops when there was really not a need. The former Eveready Bunny that I had been was now a couch sloth!

Lying down and sleeping were an escape from the confusing challenges, for sure. But also, sleep was a critical healing nutrient for my brain function. When I could, I would grab minutes here and there. You might find me in my chair, in the call room at the hospital, or even on a stretcher in the operating room waiting for my next case to start. I am probably fortunate that I was never mistakenly wheeled into surgery *myself*, waking to discover the loss of my appendix or something else! Of course, I'm kidding about the potential for mistake. I am not kidding about grabbing rest whenever and wherever I could. In many ways, it was a *strange* life!

Saturdays were the pits! I would sleep in as long as I could before getting out of bed. I would then clean up and head to the recliner. I would stay there most of the day, trying to get the "pressure" to ease off. By Saturdays, the pressure was so intense, I was miserable with it.

Ah, "pressure." "What is that?", you ask. Let me see if I can find the words. To me, pressure was different from a headache. Others might not separate the two. Some could interpret it as low-grade, constant headache. I have rarely had migraines. They are intense and difficult to overlook. The pressure, as I call it, was less intense than a migraine, but it was more pervasive. It was not accompanied by any visual disturbance, although I needed to avoid bright lights. There was no real nausea component.

Heaviness or fogginess might be other applicable terms. I could not localize it to a certain part of my head. It was a definite, strong feeling of discomfort, almost as if my skull had a new layer of insulation inserted. It gave me the impression of being tight in there! Strange, yes! I would feel so extremely uncomfortable. I felt my brain was telling me that all the activity and all the work during the week had bruised it. I needed to slow down, cool my jets, and withdraw.

It seemed to help when I limited motion, activity, and intense mental effort. My wife had me swear off the ever-present medical journals during these times. I also tried to avoid loud noises from TV, etc. Isn't it frustrating that when anytime you want to enjoy your "relaxation time," instead, you have to plan quiet, restrictive recuperation? Movies, concerts, and most other outings were literally *out*! There were many activities I deferred on those Saturdays. Boring, that is what I was! I realized I had no choice, and that can be a very defeating feeling.

Those Saturdays were difficult to overcome. As Christmas approached, on one of those Saturdays, we had to take the obligatory shopping trip to the mall. We would start with the drive. For us, that was forty-five minutes or so. Most of the road is open, but there are curves and stops and starts, of course. Then, there was the city traffic. This would set me up to be, shall we call it, a tad bit unsettled.

Mary and I walked into the mall to begin our shopping. Particularly, as this was Christmas shopping, the place was congested with other shoppers. I feel sure you can reconstruct the typical environment. There were always stores doing things to attract customers. It could be startling when several stores in a row are blaring music that may contrast with the "elevator music" found in the general mall background. The stimuli would rapidly start to get to me. Let me tell you, that is a terror-rich environment. Wow, so many stimuli! There were flashing lights, bright-colored window displays, music from multiple origins, and, of course, people talking at all loudness-levels, quickly whizzing by!

This seemed to always be worse on the second floor for me. There, in addition to what is happening right around you, you can add noise and activity coming up through the open portal between floors. I could not take it. In my world, this was all intensified to the point of being overwhelming. My senses were throbbing. I had to leave! I think what really pushed me over the top was all the movement activity. As noted, kids running past, adults shoving through, or even just the normal merging of shoppers, would push me over the top of discomfort. So many stimuli, from so many sources, and I had no perceptual filter. It got tight, and all that up-close and intense input was more than I could process and survive.

If I was going to get by, as easily as possible, in this new universe where I found myself living, I had to limit the challenging environments to which I exposed myself. One of the sources of joy that I was forced to refigure was taking trips to the beach. Walking on the beach is a multi-faceted challenge for someone with poorly-controlled vestibular symptoms.

I have been going to the beach since I was in diapers. I grew up landlocked, but the highlights of my year were beach trips to a relative's cottage in North Carolina. I walked, ran, dug, got buried, hunted shells, and rolled like a ball in the surf. Parental supervision back then was less intense. We kids helped one another. I did have my run-ins with needing to be yanked up from under the water by a bigger hand, but there was always one when I needed it! Sunburn was an annual challenge during a July 4 holiday week. After all, back then, the only sunscreen was a t-shirt. Beach joy wasn't without its price, but I loved it. I still do.

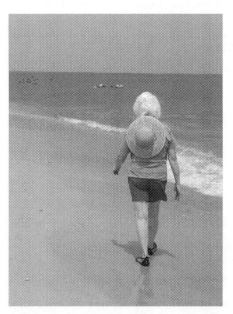

Walking the beach.

I never really questioned the beach setting. The surf can be intense, the sun bright, and the wind powerful. There are days in the winter that are overcast and stormy. I have protective rain gear, and I have cold-weather gear. I was always ready for whatever weather conditions were present. Barring a hurricane, my acceptance was universal. I would get out there under almost any conditions. "Bring it on," I would say. "God, let me see Your power!" I loved the wind and the shearing of water off the crests of the waves. But now, after the injury, that has changed. The challenges to overcome at the beach include:

1. Variable winds that may bump you from side to side, unpredictably.
2. Slanting beach where you walk with one foot stepping higher than the other. Every step tilts you left or right.
3. Sounds from the surf are inconsistent and variable in frequency and volume.
4. As you walk, you scan. You look further down the beach, then near your feet for shells, and then out to sea. As you scan, your center of gravity is simultaneously rocking from the uneven sand. All this change in distance and detail, from a rocking base, can be provocative.
5. Walking on sand that is inconsistent, sometimes collapsing under your foot, and sometimes feeling hard, sends inconsistent feedback to the brain, forcing additional processing.

Who would have thought a walk on the beach could be so challenging? All my life it had been my time to relax, reflect, and become spiritual with the Maker of the universe. Now I found myself sitting on the sand, trying to recover from losing the battle with such a multiplicity of sensory inputs. The variety of data that all through my life had thrilled me, now overwhelmed my ability for processing. My lack of filter led to data-overload and operational failure! It was sad coming to this realization.

During the time of my worst symptoms, I didn't go walking on the beach by myself. When I did go, I sometimes took a hiking stick. Walks were either avoided or disappointingly short and were often accompanied by my wife, who gave me her arm for stability. We used our special arm embrace, which was more stable and helpful for me. This is noted below.

For the first time in my life, I wanted to get off that beach! This led to timidity in even *trying* to walk on the shore. A sad situation for a lifelong beachcomber.

There were so many changes that I adopted with time. Other weekend compromises involved crowds and theaters. If I did attend a lecture or a sermon, I became like a "Back Row Baptist." The first step was always to identify the loudspeakers and triangulate the most distant point from all of them. To quote the flight attendant speech as a plane trip begins, I was always "aware of the nearest exit"!

In the early days, when I did get out and drive around town, I would sometimes get lost. Talk about scary! Here is a grown man, a professional, a longtime resident in his community, pulled over to the side of the road. I recognized where I was. What I had difficulty with figuring out was how to get from one known place to another known place. With a little time, I could usually figure it out. Or sometimes it helped to just continue to drive. But not always. There was more than once when I took advantage of that portable cell phone to call Mary and get her to guide my drive to my destination. That was certainly humiliating, embarrassing, and very disconcerting for someone who was once full of self-confidence.

Let me tell you something my wife and I developed, even if I am sure I was not the first to utilize the technique. It doesn't prevent or stop disoriented reacting, but it does help you get through your reaction. If your balance is off, you may have difficulty walking in a straight, coordinated fashion. In public, that can be embarrassing. If you are in a hallway, tracing a hand against the wall is something you can try. It's certainly something I have often done. There are times when no wall is along your path. There are some environments, such as the beach, a mall, or a trail, that are especially challenging to one's balance success. Holding hands with your spouse or friend can be helpful, but, for me, that didn't really yield a feeling of security or comfortable stability. Mary and I began the technique of bracing arms, as pictured below. In this position, there is much more contact between forearms. This leads to more stability and a feeling of security. Other observers may just think it is "sweet" and not be suspicious of a failing. I would recommend trying this when your condition requires assistance and you need to get back to your car or seat.

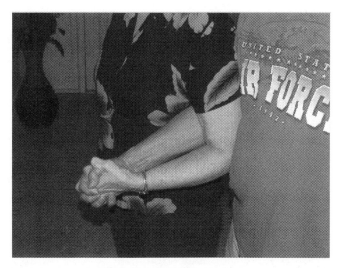

Braced arm stability hold.

I had another symptom that was so "special," it affected me as a surgeon. Those of you who haven't gone to an operating room to work, probably don't realize that we can do all kinds of things with an operating table. In addition to the up-and-down feature, you can also roll the table to the right or left and tilt the head up or head down. The most common thing that a gynecologist requires for an abdominal pelvic procedure is for the patient to be tilted head-down. That is named the Trendelenburg position. Whether operating through an incision or by laparoscopy, the head-down position makes it easier to shift more mobile parts of the internal anatomy towards the upper abdomen, creating more operating space in the pelvis.

Well, that maneuver is something I had been utilizing for years, ever since way back in my medical-school days. But now, there was a new game in town! I would be performing surgery and be proceeding just fine. Early on, at times, the anesthesia provider would make an *unannounced*, voluntary change in the table's position. He was thinking he was helping me see better! Well, let me tell you, when you have issues handling movement in your surroundings, and you have your eyes intensely fixed on a stable object, you don't *want* that table suddenly going up, down, or into a tilt! When that table moved unexpectedly, it took me for quite a disorienting, rotating, spinning ride. I would put my hands down and hold on! I was suddenly out of commission! Sometimes that unexpected trip was so rough I had to sit against the wall for a few minutes. This was a lesson I learned very early. I had to impress upon the team that such altering of the table was not acceptable.

Before you conclude that I might have been dangerous, I *always* had another surgeon with me during this time in my recovery. It did not take long before the anesthesia guy took my new status seriously. For myself, I learned that when I needed to have the table height or angle adjusted, I should look away, ask for the adjustment, and not look back until it was completed. Staring at solid walls was a lot safer! I could always look back and have the table adjusted further; I just did not have to watch it!

Maybe you will see yourself in this term: "spacey." For me, "spacey" meant my brain computing was at a standstill. It was a feeling that I had stepped out of reality, in a way, and could absorb no more input. I was adrift. As I will mention later, in connection with a run, I had to just sit and recover. When I was really "spacey," I could not meaningfully relate to others. Simple "Yes" and "No" answers were my forte. Also, I would not be as cognizant of my surroundings. My focus was inward. I had spaced out, quite effectively, and I would need time to redirect my view outwardly again.

For me, "foggy" was similar to "spacey," but not as severe. You may identify with the term "foggy" more easily. My wife would mean pretty much the same thing when she was recovering from a migraine. She would say she felt "dull." Dull and foggy are probably very similar terms for describing sensations of cognitive blunting, a perceived slowing of your ability to think and function. This type of symptom was very threatening to me. My professional life to this point, through all the academic training and testing I had endured, and through my daily clinical life, required me to be sharp and quick. Slowing was not consistent with functional. And, if it had persisted, it could have been a career-ending change!

Have you ever played word search? I do not mean a board game or a puzzle on a page. I mean, how often have you been in a conversation and the words you wish to speak just will not come?! I have had this deficiency at intervals, and it has caused me embarrassment. Give me a message which has been written down, and I can deliver it with conviction. Ask me to be spontaneous on a non-medical subject, and you may find me pausing to locate those words somewhere hidden away in my brain. The pauses usually did not happen when I was giving a programmed response. In the clinical setting, most of the answers I gave, I had already given "a thousand times." Well, maybe not that many, but I did have answers pretty well down-pat from experience and prior need. I was more at risk if I was having a random or spontaneous conversation. This was particularly true if I was reaching or stretching my knowledge base in the conversation to something I had not utilized recently. Interestingly enough, explanations of endometriosis, fibroids, or ovulation would flow freely. If, however, a friend in the office would ask about what my children were doing now, I would have to reflect and would be more prone to stumbling.

Unfortunately, this still happens for me. A recent example is that I had a painter come by the other day to discuss some potential work for us. I had called him, and I knew he was coming *sometime*, which is all the info he had offered. I guess I was not prepared when he actually walked up and knocked on the door. Even though I am pretty familiar with lingo about paint and painting, I haven't recently used it very much. When that painter was walking through the house with me, discussing what we wanted, I kept blanking on the terms I needed. I even had challenges remembering words like "ceiling" and "door frame." That can be *very* embarrassing.

A rare encounter with a painter, where words do not flow well, is one thing. What if I had been out in the evening, as I have been sometimes in the past, with a glass of wine in my hand, and I couldn't find the words? Depending on whom I was talking with, how close our relationship might be, and the nature of the occasion, there might really be a risk for starting the rumor mill. Well, that is one reason for a *one-glass* or *no-glass* policy.

So, if you feel at risk for embarrassing, word-usage difficulties, be careful how you may expose yourself to those who are not in-the-know. On the other hand, try not to withdraw unnecessarily. Hopefully, getting out on a limited basis, in the appropriate setting, will help you to build skills and confidence. As you battle for recovery, engaging with friends will help you avoid the self-pity of withdrawal. Deciding when and how to venture out is one of those times where your support person can be very instrumental. Mary hangs tight at my side when we are in new or different circumstances.

If you are reading this as a fellow sufferer, you will realize that I have exposed my self-defined inadequacies, deficiencies, weaknesses, and struggles. I have become vulnerable to my readers. Even after these years, with all my clinical experiences, and my reading on the subject, I still struggle with being unsure as to how many others have experienced such symptoms as these to such an extent. Some of my responses and feelings have been almost bizarre. For instance, when that operating table shifted quickly, I might suddenly let out a belch. Yes, a belch! The belch could also happen, instantaneously it seemed, when I was riding in a car that made an unanticipated speed change, like a sudden stop. That is the *strangest* thing. I don't understand it, I can only report it. Sometimes I wonder, how did the aliens take over this body that used to be mine?!

Let me put you in my day: Being on call, meant I could be "called" and have to respond immediately. I might be in the office, in my car, or around town. The worst, though, is being called into action in the middle of the night. Picture this! I am dead asleep. The phone rings. That hand of mine reaches out, just like it did at Wilford Hall. Now, however, that bedside table is in place. I grab the phone and hold it to my ear. "Hello," is spoken in a groggy fog. The nurse (any of whom would pretty much recognize my voice in all its forms) would start relating the situation. Sometimes, the call might be to get permission to administer a requested medicine. I say, "Okay," hang up, and usually I go immediately back to Z-land. Sometimes, that phone call would reveal something to the effect of, "Jane Doe just arrived, and she is completely dilated. You need to **get here now**!" Click! Okay, I had to hustle to get there and catch this baby! Time to jump into action! However, as you know by now, my "jumper" was defective after the fall.

You have been there. You wake up in the middle of the night due to a noise or a need to visit the bathroom. You struggle a little bit to wake up enough to sit up, and then you stay on the side of the bed, to "get your bearings." With determination, you slowly walk until you are awake enough to see to your business.

I did not have that luxury. I had to "jump start" my heart and brain, rush to get on my scrubs, hustle out the door, and speed off to Labor and

Delivery. That is a challenge even when you have all your faculties! When you are suffering vestibular dysfunction, immediate action requires amassing every potential you possess. I must admit that, as I charged out of bed, I hit a few door jambs, maybe even a direct walk into a wall or two. You could have seen me tripping, as I was trying to maintain balance, while I put one leg after another into my scrub pants. By that time, I would be waking up. I walked up the hallway with a hand against the wall and made my way out the door. The short two-mile trip to the hospital allowed me to focus my thinking and review what I was about to do. Fortunately, there is usually no traffic at 2:00 or 3:00 a.m. It is also fortunate that I was always responding to the same location. Learned and patterned responses carried me through many a challenge.

SO, WHAT WAS IT REALLY LIKE? It was disconcerting, intimidating, and scary! It was a daily uncertainty. It was confusing as to what the day would hold and what the future might encompass.

CHAPTER 8

First Clinical Steps

"Older and wiser voices can help you find the right path, if you are only willing to listen." Jimmy Buffett

It was the day of my first neurology visit. I knew this neurologist because I had previously worked with him. I had hopes he would be the guide to help me understand my new realm of experience. I will mention him more than once, for Richard Blackburn, MD, was indeed the caring and accepting physician who helped me sail these new, unchartered waters. I have worked with many neurologists over my career. Let me tell you that it seems each medical specialty has a characteristic personality. The prototype personality for a neurologist, as I see it, is that they are very cerebral, theoretical, and not generally very personable. Some might even be labeled as "different." Well, I guess we are all "different" in our own special ways. I was really different myself, especially at that first visit as Dr. Blackburn's patient!

It has been fifteen years, sailing those confusing seas, since that fateful February day. I saw Dr. Blackburn this month for what I hope will be my last visit (September, 2019). To continue the analogy, he has been the sextant that guided me along this seaway back to normalcy. I am very thankful for his patience and steadiness along the way. I am very appreciative that he accepted me as a patient in need and worked towards helping me improve. Acceptance is a big deal. To be accepted by your family, co-workers, and physician, despite how your responses have seemingly changed you, makes so much difference in being positive during the battle. When you can't fully understand or accept your own symptoms, genuine acceptance of *you*, as you *are*, by those you care about, is a real building-block to recovery.

Every time I have been to see Dr. Blackburn, he has gone through a complete neurological exam. He always checks my reflexes, my sensation to touch, my hearing, my coordination, my memory, my walk; seemingly everything neurologic. I have seen some doctors of many specialties that give you a fairly complete exam once on the first visit and never repeat it. Not so, Dr. Blackburn. I am sure that his thorough *and* consistent approach is the best way to compare and catch changes over time.

Whenever we drove down and arrived at his office, it was usually quiet in the reception room and the staff always greeted me in a friendly manner. I would get called to the back and sit on that exam table. Dr. Blackburn would enter, and we would exchange greetings. He would ask me how I was doing. I would try to be honest, but, you know, that is really a hard question to answer. You have two bad alternatives you must stay between. One of the bad choices is to list all the dysfunctional details and seem like a wimp. (Just how much time do you have, doctor? You won't believe this, but…). I refused to be wimpy or pitiful. The other bad choice is to try and fake it, putting up a tough façade. (I'm doing fine, thank you.) The second choice is bad because it hides from the doctor the depth of your need. It is also bad because he can't reliably tell if his interventions are helping you, unless you open up. I will add a third reason it is bad: it is dishonest. After all, I was in the "head doctor's office"! Duh! I would not be coming if I were "just fine." I could not really hide it all, anyway. He knew from the look in my eyes, at times, and how I walked close to the wall, that I was far from "just fine"! I needed to "fess up," but I tried to do it in a straightforward way.

Let me address that openness issue a little more. I was suffering on a daily basis, but I was also optimistic. I just kept expecting it to get better. In retrospect, I believe I actually stayed in arrested denial for a long time. I really did not understand what was happening. I just was not even considering that the new me had a long-term potential.

If the doctor started me on a new medicine to try and reduce the headaches, I just assumed it would improve things. As a doctor myself, I knew better than that. I should have kept up with some method of measurement. I could have marked headache-free or headache-bothered days on a calendar. I could have tried to analyze if the headaches were less frequent, less intense, or shorter in duration. I just did not want to become a *professional* patient with charts and diaries, etc. While I could not make myself go to that extreme, I really should have done a better job of monitoring. That would have been in my best interest because it would have given more objective information to my doctor.

I learned that to get the most out of my doctor visits, I needed to be open and report honestly. What I learned to do, and what seemed to help, was taking some time on the trip down to review the interval since the last doctor visit. That did bring to mind issues I felt needed to be addressed. It was also helpful to ask my wife, "What should I tell the doctor today?" She would help out with details and also remind me of symptoms that I had been trying to overlook or forget! The last event in his exam is always for me to walk up and down the hall while he watches my attempt at a coordinated stride. That sounds simple, does it not? Any "normal" person can walk up and down the hall, right? Well, guess what? I was not normal!

Now, these many years later, the walk is just that: a walk, a turn around, and a walk back. No big deal. Not so in the early days. For a typical visit, I would probably work right up to the time to leave for the appointment, taxing my brain. We would ride down in the car for the fifty-five-minute trip, including negotiating Tallahassee city traffic, stressing my brain further. Depending on what condition I might be in from overtaxing my brain that day and the days prior, how much sleep I had or had not gotten, and how rough the traffic was, I might be all set up to fail. It was challenging to go through the baring of my symptoms to him and I was challenged by the other physical maneuvers during his preliminary exam. I had to try and concentrate on my three-word memory test. All this effort often used up whatever reserve I had managed to maintain. By the end of that visit I was not always capable of "coordinated stride" during that last test. There was a time there when I left a trail along the wall as my hand helped to provide some stable reassurance.

Note here: My wife was doing the driving down to the visit and other times as well. That was a necessity. Before my injury, I had always done the lion's share of the driving when we were together, but that had to change. I could not handle keeping up with all the variables of cars moving in and out of lanes, etc.

No physician can be the all-in-all of everything you desire. All of us, as physicians, have our strengths and weaknesses. Once you see the doctor, you know he/she is going to order tests. I went through the CT scans, MRIs, EEGs, Sleep Studies, Balance Tests, and more exams by other specialists. I didn't perform too sporty on the balance tests, but all of the hard-imaging, such as the CT and MRI, came back "normal." Looking back, I wanted to understand what was happening and I wanted medical help to resolve my symptoms. I did not really understand why the imaging came back normal. I sure did not feel normal. It took me a while to really appreciate that the damage I had experienced was on the cellular level. My injury involved supposed disruptions of neuron activity and cell-to-cell communication. That level of injury just does not show up on the routine imaging which you get with a standard MRI or CT scan.

In addition, I was really seeking out validation as part of the medical interaction. My world had been rocked! I wanted someone to say, "I understand!" I wanted a trained professional to say, "I recognize this, you have _____." It would even be reassuring to hear, "This is all secondary to the fall. It may not be common for these symptoms to persist like this, but it has happened in others and now it has happened in you. It is real. We will try to help you." Another reassurance I looked for, because I was experiencing such bizarre, activity-altering symptoms, was somebody to say, "You are sane!" It would be nice for your physician to say something to the effect of, "I have never been where you are, and I don't fully understand, but I do respect the battle you are waging." Validation can be the first step toward forming a physician-patient team bond. While we would like for the doctor to immediately cure our ills, many times that is not possible. It certainly is not true with head injury.

To be objective, it is necessary to realize that if the doctor has never dealt with you before, and if your studies come back "normal," he/she may take a little while to really understand what is happening and what is causing your symptoms. Certainly, some patients do go off the deep end malingering, and some do have psychiatric issues. Other patients, clinicians realize, are looking for a way to get out of work and onto benefits. As patients, we have to allow the medical team to analyze and gain familiarity with our story and symptoms. As struggling patients who are fighting for improvement, somewhere along the way we long for a hand on the shoulder, a statement of validation, or a commitment to stay the course with us. These assurances can go a long way toward building trust and comfort.

Let me tell you about some of the steps I went through to analyze my condition. When I saw Dr. Blackburn for the first time, he was alerted to the distress I was experiencing. I was having memory issues. I was having difficulty concentrating. We called it "cognitive dysfunction." That just means my "thinker" wasn't working at its best. Once again, I was scared. I was afraid that I might not be as good at doing my job as I needed to be. As a physician, I could not afford to not give my best, defined as my pre-injury best! Patient-care required my being sharp and capable. There could be no compromising a patient's future health because my current abilities might be altered.

I am sure that feeling of needing to be your best is true in many professions and occupations. I would not want someone working with electricity or fixing my roof who was not fully aware and in control. All of us need to feel capable and confident in our own areas of experience and expertise. I think that is especially true for moms caring for their babies, where every day is a training day, and one must be sharp to keep check on new talents the kiddos develop overnight!

Memory is often a part of the initial set of challenges in the cognitive behavior category. It is also one of those really difficult areas to assess. It is difficult for each of us to be objective about our own qualities of memory. And it is also difficult for professionals to accurately diagnose subtle memory issues. Somewhere between the four-year-old, who remembers every bad word you ever said, and the elderly sufferer of dementia, there is a large area of variation in what most of us realize we remember.

We have all heard of the rare victim that suffers from amnesia. More commonly, each of us can suffer from difficulty in two primary areas of memory: short-term and long-term. While I will not write a discourse on the function and division of memory, I will use my working understanding. We file away important facts from our past, such as memories of our weddings, what our kids looked like as babies, and where we have lived. I still know my street address for my childhood home, for instance. That was fifty years ago now. This collection of memories from the past is generally classified as long-term memory. Our more functional memory, also called short-term memory, helps us remember more day-to-day needs and changes. Short-term memory is required when we need to take a casserole out of the oven at a certain time. It helps us to remember where we parked our car at the mall. And it helps us to compare prices at the grocery store.

For some reason, most of us men would declare that women have the best long-term memory mechanism. Women are the ones who remember wedding dates best, remember Aunt Clara's birthday, and may be better able to describe that first date you shared. This is, of course, a generality. We men do come up with old memories, as well. What we are best at remembering may have to do with our value systems. Guys, you probably do not need help to remember the biggest fish you ever caught. You can remember the big buck you shot. You recall who your buddies were in school. You just may have more difficulty pinning an actual date on these items.

Short-term memory is where most people find their difficulty. This is true of our elders, but it is also true during recovery from a concussion. You, no doubt, have seen cartoons about elders walking into a different room in the house, then forgetting why they made the journey. That can be humorous and entertaining from afar, but it can also be disturbing when it happens to us personally! Once in a while, if we forget why we walked into another room, we can write it off and not get too concerned. But distress is especially common if we feel it is happening repeatedly. Short-term memory talent does slowly degrade over the years. Memory exercises may help to keep you stronger in your abilities here.

It is interesting that in my case, what alerted me initially to my concussion symptoms was seemingly a memory issue. In actuality, what I couldn't bring forward was an event that was fixed in my long-term memory. That is the area that is supposed to be more resistant to injury. My conclusion is that memory was not really the problem that day! While I would struggle with short-term memory in the days to come, my issue that first day was a generalized slowing of my brain responses. Due to a disturbance in cognitive, higher-level function, I was failing at pulling the data forward.

Let me put you in the shoes I was in. The modern-day doctor is supposed to take his/her computer into the room and input information into the record as he/she is asking questions. That will work, but most patients would rather look for caring in the eyes of the physician, as opposed to scanning a black laptop lid with a maker's mark. Way back when I was trained, we called it "taking a history." That is what I still call it. The more modern term is "data collection." That data collection, with the nurse or physician seemingly hiding from view, can come across as very impersonal. I could never do that laptop thing simultaneously with talking. My method always had to be this way: sit, converse, and ask the pertinent questions that I needed answered. I looked in the eyes and I read body language. That is what patients preferred, but it is also what made me feel more involved and compassionate. It gave me clues when a patient said one thing with her mouth, but her eyes related there was more to be told.

The challenge, though, has always been to remember those details when later recording the visit. This is not a new problem. Retaining those important clinical facts is essential. This was true in the days when notes were primarily dictated. It is still true today, when it is typically the doctor's requirement to complete the "electronic record" before the patient leaves. It has been, and will continue to be, critical to get those facts recorded correctly. (By the way, that "finishing the electronic record before the patient leaves" is also a story for another day or may be better termed a fantasy for another day.)

Once I would leave the exam room, while the patient was getting ready for an exam or a procedure, or once I had completed the visit with the patient, I needed to remember the details until I could find the time to record them. Failing to record that data accurately can be a big oversight and it is something most of us take very seriously. For instance, I would need to remember what she said she was using for birth control, I would need to remember how long she said her periods lasted, and I would need to remember her problems and the details of her pain. If I failed to record accurate and clinically significant information, it would be lost forever.

Of course, not documenting all this information can create difficulties and oversights during the current visit, such as confusion about what prescriptions were written. Also, during future visits, I or another clinician should review the note being recorded today. Leaving out pertinent facts, or getting confused and recording inaccurate information, may steer the original physician, or another, down the wrong path of questions in any future encounter. This potentially could degrade the patient's care for multiple visits to come, over months and even years. It is a disservice to the patient to not be accurate and complete. The patient has higher expectations from her professional caregiver! She deserves expert-level care, as well as accurate recording.

Memory function is a constant need for all of us throughout our day. Have you forgotten to get a gas fill-up before you ran out? Have you forgotten to pick up that bread or milk you promised you would bring home? Did you forget and leave the roast in the oven until it was leather? My late mother-in-law was always needing her glasses and always forgetting where she left them. I do not know how many searches I have undertaken in that quest. Personally, I can't ever remember where I have left my coffee cup.

You see, we all have memory challenges and memory failings. It is just part of our daily challenge. I think most of the day-to-day memory problems we have are based on distractions in our environment. Our fast-paced world has zoomed us into a reality that often forces us to "multi-task." In fact, we often pride ourselves on the number of tasks we are keeping up with simultaneously, comparable to one of those stage acts where they keep multiple plates spinning on sticks.

As for me, for better or worse, I have always multi-tasked. In my profession, this was not a matter of choice. Often, while I was seeing a patient in the office, I was also on alert for a patient in labor or for a post-operative patient. Some would say this multi-task thing can be defined as doing multiple things poorly at the same time. Unfortunately, that may indeed often be true. To multi-task successfully in areas of critical importance requires a high level of intellectual intensity and effort! We must all accept some of this overlapping activity as the culture we live in currently. We have to be careful to not slight areas of significance, in the distraction caused by background chatter.

When you are at home, how often do you concentrate on one activity at the time? Don't you have the T.V. on or have background music playing? Aren't you checking your text messages, emails from family or the office, and social media pages? Isn't all this happening while you are trying to relate to your family, reading, doing cooking or housework, playing with the dog, or completing a project? When you think about it, memory distraction must be legit. It is responsible for the plethora of timers in our homes. We have timers on the stove and the microwave. We have automatic turn-offs for space heaters and coffee pots. Some of us set chimes on our watches to keep up with the hours as they pass or set alarms to avoid overlooking a meeting or pick-up time. If such "forgetfulness" was not common, would we really find timers everywhere? You are not alone, my friend!

When you leave in the morning, you take more with you than what you chose to wear. You also take with you plans for the workday, plans for picking up kids, plans for meals, plans for a hundred things seemingly. You may also take a few moments to look ahead to consider, "How do I get away on a vacation?" We are blessed with active minds, and we can manage to simultaneously keep many issues straight. Don't give yourself too hard a time when you fail at remembering a detail here or there.

When I was in the deepest throes of trying to gain control after my head injury, I had a big issue with concentration. I looked back at my pre-injury life. I labeled my former self as a "highly functional individual." I expected to be able to remember details and keep track of multiple high-level issues simultaneously. When I left that exam room, I felt I better remember the details, or I was letting my patient down. But, after the injury, there was a new order of things. When I was walking next to the wall for stability and having to sit down occasionally to regain spin control, it was very distracting, as you can imagine. Those efforts did affect my ability to focus and to concentrate. Others who have fallen prey to concussion sequelae can probably easily identify with my challenge here. I had to find helps!

Dr. Blackburn started me on a medicine called memantine hydrochloride, which is generally used on patients suffering from Alzheimer's disease. "It is something we can try," he suggested. He thought it would be helpful. Let me tell you, being fifty-three years of age with a wife and two kids, and being offered a medicine used for dementia, that will get your attention. Fortunately, this part of my dysfunction cleared up much quicker than some of the other symptoms.

In addition to taking medication, I also picked up a pad and paper. I learned my own shorthand for keeping important info in my "peripheral memory." It was not nearly as divisive between the patient and myself as a computer would be. Since I used abbreviations, it did not really take much writing to provide the clues I would later expand on in the note. That same trick is something I have recommended over and over again to my patients. Why beat up on yourself over presumed memory deficits? If you feel you have a medical issue or that you are far worse off than others, seek medical evaluation and help. I did! You may have a problem than can be helped clinically. For most of us, including me now, we are somewhere in the land of variation called "normal." For us, it is down to trying to figure out a way to get by efficiently. After all, do you go to the grocery store without a shopping list? Most people do not. Those who do go without a list, I am told, spend more money due to random grabbing, especially if they are hungry at the time of shopping.

For years, I have kept a pad by my bed. Rather than stay awake wondering if I will remember an issue of importance for the next morning, I just write it down. This dates back to before my last injury. It allows me to not occupy my mind and to rest better, while being assured to not overlook the issue after I arise. Notes can also be helpful in remembering what errands you need to run or what tasks you need to accomplish over the weekend. Some people use dry erase boards, sticky notes, etc., for such aides. We all lead busy lives; do not hold yourself in contempt over an impossible standard. It is discouraging to feel like you are failing; do not set yourself up to let it continue. Develop and work your system!

Dr. Chrisanne Gordon informs me that one of the medicines used now to help promote post-concussion function is amantadine. I am familiar with using this drug to treat the flu. In neurology, it is also used to help manage patients with Parkinson's disease. It may enhance the function of dopamine in certain tissues, improving nerve communication and function. I am sure there are other medicines and therapies that I am not currently aware of. My list here is based on my experiences and is not meant to be any type of comprehensive guide. Your best bet for help is to find a caring professional with talent and experience, who is up to date in this field.

Another especially important aspect of staying under control is to build your team around you. My wife knows I just will not remember some things. That was true, of course, even before my head trauma. Sometimes that "whole two-mile trip" to work would take me out of the home world, transfer me into the clinical world, and wipe my memory clean like that dry-erase board I mentioned. In fact, if she desired for me to do something or to try to remember something, until I reached the office, she just sent me an email that would come up and remind me while I was at my desk. It helped! I am also very thankful for my office assistant at the time, Kathy Johnson. Kathy served to get patients to the exam rooms, take vital signs, prepare for exams and procedures, chaperone the patient encounter, and assist in any way needed. Those needs certainly increased after my fall. She came through in a thoroughly caring way and was very impactful in my recovery. I will always be thankful for her understanding and assistance. Like my wife, she could tell when my symptoms were winning. She helped me plan my day, helped to make sure I remembered items of importance, and was, most of all, accepting and patient with me. That understanding, acceptance, and comprehensive assistance was a key component in my being able to continue to function at a high level.

My team was responsible for keeping my function at the standard of excellence I demanded. I cannot stress enough how important it is to be able to be open and honest with those closest to you. You need love and caring. You need facilitators. You need supportive people who are looking for ways to ease your challenges. One of the particularly essential benefits from such a team is encouragement. Each day is frustrating when you compare the "what I am" with the "what I was." I could even express it as a grief response. I will talk about that later. The members of your team must be a small, trustworthy, and confidential group.

Those of us affected are having a hard-enough time accepting our current limitations. Most of us feel very uncomfortable with being an "open book" describing brain dysfunction or even transient, mental-function limitations to others. In addition to surrounding yourself with supporters, it is so very helpful to have at least one inner-circle confidant. To heal and to maintain perspective, I feel we must share the distress and frustration we experience with our most trustworthy intimate.

As I have mentioned, I have served as a professional who lived in a small town of under 13,000. This is the first time I have really gone public with the severity of the battle I waged and the challenges I endured. I required a lot more rest, and that curtailed some of my activities. I was also motivated to limit my extra-curricular activities to obscure the opportunity that others might witness one of my struggles.

We all celebrate Saturdays. It is a day when most of our work schedules permit us to have some freedom to pursue projects, leisure, and fun. For a long time after the last concussion, I remember Saturdays weren't really the Saturdays of old. It was no longer a day where I could work or play outside, go off, enjoy sports, or pursue other options. Traveling was especially off the table. This curtailed my presence and activity in the community. I no longer would participate in helping to clean our waterways or go to local craft fairs. I had to withdraw. During that season of challenge, those years, the typical Saturday was almost totally committed to rest. I would rest my head: the best solution/treatment I ever discovered for those times when the symptoms were overpowering. In the early days, by the time Saturday rolled around, the symptoms were always overpowering!

SO, WHAT WAS IT REALLY LIKE? Have you ever been all dressed up with your shoes shined and your hair combed? Ladies, you know what it is like to build your image before a formal occasion. Between the right clothing, the make-up, and the hair style, you can project the image you desire for people to see; you can impact their perception of you, even as you may improve your perception of yourself.

Having to open up about strange, weird, and unexplainable symptoms is akin to ripping off all that façade. It is like being naked: exposed for all to evaluate and criticize, as they choose. That is what it is like to open up after a head injury as you try to survive the day-to-day disorder. It's embarrassing, disturbing, and potentially humiliating as you admit your "failings." Even so, it is necessary in order to start the trip back to normalcy!

CHAPTER 9

Headaches

"He that is good at making excuses is seldom good for anything else." Benjamin Franklin

I did deal with headaches. They were just never severe to the point that I considered them one of my bigger issues. I never got much response using ibuprofen or naproxen. Acetaminophen was my best help, when I was bothered to the point of wanting a relief aid. My doctor wanted to help me with those headaches by putting me on medicine as a preventative. There are generally three steps in the plan of attack for headaches. These options are most appropriate for severe, life-disturbing headaches, primarily migraines. For a time after a significant concussion, headaches can be a real issue of distraction. Control can be essential to achieving functional focus.

If the headaches are frequent, the first step is to try a preventative medicine that you take daily. You can judge its success by an increase in headache-free days. Such a medicine can be very instrumental in the first healing stages after mild traumatic brain injury. The second step, when the first step does not achieve adequate control, is to use an abortive agent. The first real drug in this category was sumatriptan. Taking an abortive agent when you first realize a severe headache is coming on may stop it before it becomes disabling. If after thirty minutes (or up to two hours, depending on the drug) you are functioning well and experiencing relief, that is a success. If steps one and two fail, the third level is usually a narcotic pain medicine, maybe accompanied by medicine for nausea.

Having to go to the third step generally results in the loss of a day from the pain and then the lethargy of the drug therapy. Avoiding that third step is considered winning: a victory in the headache battle. In most sufferers healing from a mild traumatic brain injury, step one can be successful, without having to go further.

For me, I never had that severe a problem with pain. I tried the preventative agents and used acetaminophen when I felt it was needed. One of the most common preventative agents is gabapentin. This is a great drug. It is very safe and can be used in a wide range of dosages. It can block all kinds of false or excessive messages that your brain sends and receives. It can also help prevent headaches. It is used a lot in helping to block excess discomfort associated with chronic pain, such as that found in leg and other neuropathies. I could not really stay on it long enough to see if it helped. It may work well for some with similar symptoms, but it intensified my foggy feeling, and I soon had to stop it.

Another agent that I have used quite often in my own practice, was one that Dr. Blackburn started me on. It is called nortriptyline. Originally, this drug was designed to be an anti-depressant. It is not used for that much these days. However, it has found a new niche. In much smaller doses, it can also provide relief from excess or false pain signals. I tolerated nortriptyline successfully and it did help for a while. I stopped it down the road of recovery after my headaches were not as bothersome. Fortunately, the reactive headaches I had after the injury were some of the first symptoms to improve.

I was learning, though. Headaches are not all head "aches," after all. The way I look at it now, a headache can be a sign of some disturbance in your brain, usually of no long-term consequence. There are many other brain disturbances that can occur, that are not marked by a recognition of pain. As a clinician, I was trained that migraines were headaches of a special severity. In light of the growth of understanding over time, I have now learned there is such a thing as a non-headache, non-pain, migraine. Migraine is a diagnosis that encompasses a large variety of clinical symptoms. My new concept of migraine is that it is a label for episodic brain dysfunction. The concept of a migraine causing pain is accurate in most circumstances and may represent vascular spasms in the brain. There is even a category of migraine that fairly accurately describes my bouts: the vestibular migraine. As I became aware of this variant, I became aware of a new term, "migraine-related phenomenon." According to www.hopkinsmedicine.org, the patient-friendly information site for Johns Hopkins University, vestibular migraine "can cause vestibular symptoms with or without an actual headache. There is almost always a history of motion sensitivity since childhood, and migraine headaches at some point in the person's lifetime, even if they last occurred decades ago."

Vestibular symptoms cover a wide range of problems, including: vertigo, feeling dizzy, nausea with movement, and, for me, "spinning." My physician suggested this diagnosis. After thought and investigation, I did personally adopt that term as a way to understand part of my issues. Unfortunately, giving part of my clinical symptoms a name did not really define how often I would suffer symptoms or how long episodes might last. It was as if these "migraines" were times of intensity on top of a constant background of dysfunction. I also did not find that the medicines that might suppress headaches, helped in any way to block my motion symptoms. Why the head trauma set me off on this dysfunction is one of the mysteries of brain function and dysfunction. It took me a long time to wake up to what was a fact for me: that my dysfunction was not going to just simply resolve and go away. I realized there would be baseline dysfunction punctuated by times of increased disorder. I was to spend years in the suffering.

As I have pondered my symptoms, namely my spatial insecurity, spinning, and balance issues, I have really grown in appreciation for God's creation. Our control center is the brain. It is protected by an almost rock-hard case filled with absorbing fluid (skull and cerebrospinal fluid). Hard blows can cause shifting, even within this protective skull, and produce injury. Fortunately, most blows do not really have a significant effect. When concussion does occur, it is based upon potential coup and contrecoup forces. This means that the brain is impacted at the site of the blow (coup), but it is also potentially impacted at the opposite side of the skull (contrecoup) when the brain bounces or shifts within its skull housing in response to the velocity imposed by the hitting force. Therefore, concussion can result in injury in more than just the area of direct impact.

The particular blow I sustained in my most recent fall was a direct impact to the back of my head, the area referred to as the occiput. The brain lying just under the occiput is labeled the occipital cortex and functionally is termed the visual cortex. This is certainly not the only area of the brain that helps to accomplish vision, but it is the major center for visual perception and coordination. The opposite pole of the brain is the frontal lobe, and just below that area lie the eyes. The frontal lobe is often associated with emotions.

Have you ever considered the miracle of vision and visual memory? The eyes are masterpieces of divine creativity. It is amazing how we see! You know, in all my medical education, from anatomy classes to autopsies, I have never seen a brain that had any recognizable pictures stored in its folds. So, how are images stored; how does that miracle work? We can retrieve the thought of a person and their visual likeness can appear in our mind. Where does that come from? And how does it form in our consciousness? Well, the truth is that our visual abilities and our memories of visual experiences are all due to carefully orchestrated chemical reactions among the cells of the brain. We store and retrieve data through these chemical changes in our brain cells. That seems impossible to believe, except we have all experienced the reality! Can't you really see that last sunset you witnessed at the beach, in all its colors? We know the truth of what we see! We know it happens, even if *how* it happens is above the level of our comprehension. I can visualize Mary in my mind only because God has created such a complex system of chemical reactions and cellular communication! Computer programming is one level of complexity, but it is a mere, poor shadow of the Master's programming!

Each of our eyes contains approximately 125,000,000 light-reacting cells. There are two types. One type, called rods, makes up the majority of the cells. The smaller group, called cones, is centered in the middle of your visual acuity. These help us to interpret colors. We are talking here about the eye ball, a spherical structure about the diameter of a quarter, with millions and millions of cells accepting light data. Each of those cells has a direct connection to the back of your brain where the data is compiled into images. That means that these infinitesimal connections in your eye lead to infinitesimal connections with brain cells in the back of your head, where all the data is made useful.

WOW, ONLY GOD COULD DO THAT!

How do I explain the dysfunction of my injury? It makes sense to me that there could be multiple micro-injuries in the type of concussion I suffered. This could include disruption of micro-connections impacting the eye itself, or more likely even, the micro-connections in the visual cortex under the site of impact at the back of my head. We have not yet touched on how the inner ear can also be impacted by a blow. We will discuss later the disruption of calcium crystals that generally top the microcilia in the inner ear, the key area for balance. Following the actual blow, part of the body's response to any injury is to produce swelling. As the individual impacted cells struggle or die, theoretically, fluid accumulates in microscopic amounts. The loss of cells and the stretching of intracellular connections makes brain fine tuning a challenge. This process may be one of the reasons that symptoms can worsen over the first few weeks. No wonder you feel *confused* and *disoriented*!

If we depend upon the front of our brain for emotional control, at least to some degree, bruising it might lead to poorly-controlled emotions; I had that. If we depend on the visual cortex for image processing, bruising it might lead to visual confusion; I had that. If we depend on the calcium crystals on the microcilia in the middle ear for balance and stability, knocking some of those loose might lead to balance issues; I had that. All of these "minor" injuries are common with head injury and unfortunately, so are the symptoms of dysfunction.

One of the theories of vestibular migraine, whether it is the result of trauma or not, is that there is confusion of input from what the eyes see vs. what the balance mechanism of the ear senses. This mismatch leads to defects in interpretation and to balance challenges. From my explanation, it is fairly reasonable to anticipate that blows to the head could result in simultaneous spatial and balance challenges, such as I experienced. Since my visual mechanism was injured as well as my balance mechanism, I had potentially two sources of inaccurate data input and processing. Whether you call it a migraine or not, the result was that my head was not working like original equipment! Spatial confusion was real!

I remember one particularly pig-headed stance of mine. I did not want to, and would not allow myself to, realize there could be triggers that were making my time with symptoms worse. Triggers are well known in the migraine world. Just because I was not having terrible pain, did not mean that the triggers were not actively contributing to my weird symptoms associated with vestibular migraines and background dysfunction. Common triggers include: dietary elements, lack of sleep, stress, and emotional crises. Physical events, like missing meals or being subjected to motion (in the case of those with the vestibular component), can also be provocative. Migraines, as an entity, can be hormonally related to a woman's menstrual cycle as well. Others suffer from increased frequency of migraines seasonally as their allergy and sinus symptoms become more bothersome.

Motion definitely could set me off. But there were triggers in my diet, as well. It would be difficult, nigh unto impractical, to try excluding all foods that might be triggers. Food triggers will be different for different people. Lists of potential trigger foods are available from many sources. Common foods on many lists are smoked meats, aged cheeses, chocolate, and nuts. There are some common categorizations among the foods that one can watch for and begin to test by limitation.

For me, I identified numerous dietary triggers that made my symptoms worse. It was tough to give up barbecue and smoked meats, but it helped! It was not so tough for me to give up red wine, when I noted a single glass caused "pressure." A glass of white wine was usually not a problem. Certain processed meats can be triggers, but I never really identified packaged meats to be a provoker for me. I learned the hard way that a spice called tarragon was on my NO list. We were at a nice restaurant. I ordered a beautiful piece of Mahi Mahi, cooked to perfection. It was strongly flavored with this spice I was not personally familiar with at the time. I didn't really care for the flavor of the tarragon, and it seemed to reek of it. I made myself tolerate the spice because I could not see wasting that beautiful piece of fish. My cost, as a result, was the pricey bill plus three days of lost activity! Boy, the pressure hit me hard that time! I haven't knowingly touched anything with tarragon since.

My worst loss was peanuts. I live in South Georgia. The southeastern Alabama and southwestern Georgia areas comprise the peanut capital of the world. Decatur County, in which Bainbridge is located, has more acres of irrigation than any other county in Georgia, according to one survey. Much of that irrigation results in bounteous quantities of peanuts.

By coincidence, I have had a life-long love affair with the peanut in pretty much all its uses. Boiled peanuts, peanut brittle, peanut butter, cheese crackers with peanut butter, mixed nuts, etc.; I loved them all. One of my favorite ways to enjoy them was to sit in a chair at the beach with a big bag of dry-roasted peanuts, munching and contemplating. Dry-roasted peanuts are also a mainstay at baseball games, circuses, and other outdoor events. They may create some flaky mess, but they are not sticky and don't soil your clothes. You just stand up and brush off the debris. Just my style. This was the last food I wanted to give up and was, actually, the last food I did give up. My symptoms really did begin to improve when I eliminated the dry-roasted peanuts. I guess the peanuts were having their revenge! All that time I suffered before facing up to stopping intake of peanuts, they were getting even with me for all I have eaten throughout my life! The peanuts won!

A big factor in why peanuts were an issue, probably had to do with the quantity of nuts I ingested at the time! I would be covered in fragments of shell and peanut skins. It was a veritable peanut massacre! The other factor was probably my choice in peanut products. Peanuts contain some amount of tyramine. Tyramine is a naturally-occurring ingredient found in many trigger foods and may actually be the most indicted agent of trouble. The level of tyramine can increase with the age of the food. I don't know, but I suspect shelf life of roasted peanuts can be a long time. I further suspect, but cannot know for sure, that was part of the issue. I likely overate rather aged peanuts. And that may have been detrimental to my wellness. Tyramine is also present in cheeses in varying degrees. It may be, for you, that some cheeses are more tolerable than others.

All I can say, for sure, is that eliminating peanuts was one of the steps that helped reduce my symptoms. After I had finally stopped the peanuts, I felt a relief of the pressure in my head. That meant less hours and less days of dysfunction, or conversely and more optimistically, I gained hours and days of normalcy and comfort. That was quite a reward. After many years now, I haven't picked up another peanut!

You may need to survey your diet. Do you enjoy a food that is on a trigger list? You may want to pick out one food to eliminate for a few weeks and see if you feel better. If after a month there is no difference, try avoiding another food and go back to enjoying the first one you excluded.

Over time, you may find a real improvement from eliminating one of those food sources. You may find some assistance in this area in one of the resources I have listed: www.neuropt.org.

As time went by for me and my efforts at dietary controlled continued, we also pursued other therapies. Even though I had failed to get a lot of benefit out of nortriptyline, we didn't give up medical control. The next drug I was prescribed was pregabalin. This drug is advertised on TV as helping with pain from diabetic neuropathy. It can help to block those impulses from the nerves that are firing inappropriately due to the diabetic disease and damage. We all understand pain in certain ways. Pain is a necessary, protective mechanism that helps us to prevent damaging our body. However, not all pain messages are accurate reflectors of the need for warning. With some disease conditions, pain messages can be sent in excess of need and can actually be contrary to need. Diabetic foot pain is one of those, migraines are another, and, in my work, chronic bladder and pelvic pain in my patients was another. Medicines (like nortriptyline, gabapentin, and pregabalin) can ease suffering in those with chronic pain, when that pain cannot otherwise be easily alleviated.

Even though I did not suffer from chronic pain or even daily headaches, I did run through times of frequent headaches. More than that, I suffered from excessive and confusing brain messages in response to the world around me. Pregabalin was effective for me. In my way of thinking, the blocking medicines, like pregabalin in my case, help to tamp down misdirected, aberrant messages. In my conception, I can visualize multiple nerves firing, some from the center of the problem and some from the periphery. The blockers curtail these surrounding, often fuzzy, peripheral messages, allowing the message from the center, (which is the truest of the messages), to come in more clearly. This is what your brain does naturally as it filters perceptions. And it is what my brain was deficient in doing at the time. A basic way of relating this is: the simpler and more direct the input, the simpler and more direct the response.

We began the pregabalin at one dose and then increasingly adjusted it until I was under better control. It has helped me to enjoy the world around me! My symptoms became less bothersome and were much improved. The components of both medicine and time helped me to get my Saturdays back. For that I have been thankful. I was not under full control, my symptoms did not disappear, but we made progress, and that gave me hope. A rapid movement in an unexpected direction, a stop-and-go drive, or some unexpected close, visual input (such as someone cutting close walking around a corner) could still set me off. The dysfunctional response wasn't as bad and didn't last as long, but it was still difficult. Now, fifteen years later, I have finally been able to wean off that medicine. My timeline to healing has been long. But healing has come. Maybe that will encourage you to believe that, with more time, you will become more tolerant and more functional. If you are not there yet, such improvement is my prayer for you!

> SO, WHAT WAS IT REALLY LIKE? Even though head "pain" was not a big issue for me, head "dysfunction" was. It took some understanding and maturing for me to realize that the pain and dysfunction were just different faces for the same problem and that any remedy would possibly impact both. To find control, I had to be open to interventions, however they were cloaked.

CHAPTER 10

Higher Level Evaluation and Care

"By experience, we find out a short way by a long wandering." Roger Ascham

Well, I have shared with you that I went to the orthopedist for help with my back. You would think that I might have gotten some x-rays of my back. Well, no. He only wanted to get help for my head. Being about three weeks out from my injury, this visit probably coincided with the peak of my growing difficulties. The orthopedist, Dr. Dewey, did what any good doctor would do. He helped answer my need, even if I did not understand what I really needed or how to ask for it. I am thankful that he routed me in a helpful direction.

Over time, I had tests and more tests. All my bloodwork was just fine and normal. I was never determined to have any underlying new disease. My problems were all due to trauma. But the big question in my mind was, how do you find the site of the injury and put a "band-aid" on it?

I had more than one CT scan along the way. CT, or computer tomography, uses low-intensity x-ray beams released in a circular, progressive fashion. The beams record signals differently when they encounter the varying density of tissues in the body. The computer then constructs images from all the individual shots. Once the images are completed, you have black-and-white pictures that look as if the body was sawed into slices! Depending on what needs to be visualized, certain agents, or dyes, that show up in the x-rays, can be used to enhance the images. That is why a patient may receive something to drink or something through the IV before the scan. The radiologist can also zero-in on an area by making the virtual "slices" move closer together. CT scans are good for identifying larger tumors, skull impacting injuries, or internal brain bleeding, amongst other conditions. What CT scans are not good at, is seeing small, sheering injuries that tear neurons, like those found in concussions. My CTs were normal. Good; I did not have any worrisome surprises. The normal CT images helped to confirm the diagnosis of concussion and post-concussion syndrome, with which I was labeled.

I also had more than one MRI, or magnetic resonance imaging. The MRI uses radio waves and strong magnets, as opposed to x-rays. The images are generally more detailed and life-like than those from the CT scan. Contrast or dyes may be used here, as well. Generally, the imaging takes longer to perform, and the price is significantly higher. That is why you may have trouble getting an MRI approved by your insurance company. MRIs can show smaller lesions and more vascular detail. There are scanners, more likely to be found in research settings, that can actually track brain function. However, the common MRIs performed for concussion patients do *not* show brain function. And they do not show the *injuries* of minor brain trauma or concussions. Fortunately, my scans were negative.

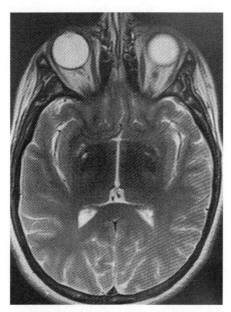

MRI image slices of human brain

Along the way, I had an EEG or electroencephalogram. The EEG picks up the electrical activity in your brain through multiple leads temporarily glued in place. EEGs are primarily used to detect seizure activity. There are multiple types of seizures. There is even one called absence or petit mal. That type of seizure may result in a short "freezing" of response from the sufferer. There are similarities in behavioral response between one person who's experiencing a petit mal seizure and another person who's experiencing the sensation I call "spacey." An outside observer may not be able to tell the difference. Investigating for that type of seizure through an EEG may help to better define your condition, help to direct your treatment, and increase your chances of symptom control.

Have you had a sleep study? I have. What a strange thing that is! They put a few EEG leads on your head, combined with straps around your chest, and they attach EKG leads for your heart. To keep up with your oxygen level, they will utilize a finger probe, as well. Once they have you all set up, they put you in a strange bed and say something to the effect of, "Sleep well." Ha! Fortunately, sleep studies have now progressed so that screening studies can be done in your home. If you suffer from certain types of sleep disturbance, it can certainly impact your daily function. Checking for sleep disorders is reasonable.

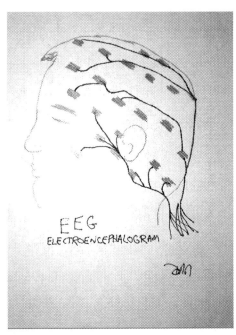

EEG leads in place.

I had other tests as parts of physician exams. We'll get to those next. Dr. Blackburn referred me for a consultation appointment to a sub-specialist in Tallahassee. This doctor, a neuro-ophthalmologist, was Dr. Charles Maitland. He was responsible for what he had labeled the Balance Disorders Clinic. As I knew him, he was the regional source for evaluation and management of patients who were suffering with stability issues. I had previously referred patients to him and have done so since my personal visit as a patient. I found him to be a kind and caring professional. He reviewed my symptoms, gave me a complete neurological exam, and then came up with a diagnosis and a plan. He spent a good bit of time talking about my inner ear. He described the workings of the inner-ear vestibular apparatus. He talked about how the calcium crystals can be disrupted or torn loose, to varying degrees, from the microcilia at the base. Those crystals can then fall into the semi-circular canals, disrupting the balance function and leading to many of the symptoms I experienced. For appropriate patients, there are maneuvers that can be done in the office or even at home to help clear these canals and improve the symptoms. The most common maneuver is called the Epley.

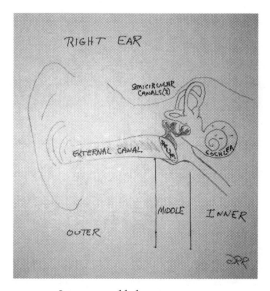

Inner ear and balance structures.

I do not know if Dr. Maitland gave me a more detailed explanation than usual, due to my baseline medical training. I do know that he put me through the same exams, tests, and careful assessment, as he would any patient presenting with similar challenges. Neither he nor his therapist ever offered the Epley maneuver to me. I know that in appropriate sufferers, it can be very helpful.

To confirm his impression, Dr. Maitland set me up for further testing in the office. There was one test maneuver he performed that was later repeated by his therapist. It was also repeated every time I went to any balance specialist. It was the Dix-Hallpike test. That particular test involves the patient, me, sitting on the table while the examiner held my head and guided me to quickly lie backwards onto the exam table until my head was just over the edge below horizontal. This would be repeated with my head facing each side. This was generally done with the examiner watching my eyes. The more "high-class" testing was done while I was wearing goggles with cameras that actually displayed my eyes on the TV monitor. The experts all took great interest in this test. Being the lowly patient, I was not always told how my eyes reacted. The best I could analyze it, based on the responses and planned steps thereafter, my test results were positive for nystagmus some of the time and negative other times.

I also had different outcomes on the caloric stimulation test. That is a test where cold water, warm water, air, or all in turn, are run into your ears. This is done on one side and then the other. This apparently is supposed to provoke nystagmus and vestibular dysfunction when they exist in the patient. At one point, I had no response and was told I had inner-ear damage. At another time, in another office, I was told my inner ear was working correctly. Their explanation for the contrary result was that I must have just had ear wax the first time. My point here is that any testing that tries to evaluate functions within your skull is difficult. Make sure you evaluate your evaluators. Determine where you will place your trust. Trust will be very important if your symptoms and dysfunction drag out for years, and the trail becomes a long one.

Let me tell you, those guys can come up with some bizarre testing. In an adjacent area to Dr. Maitland's clinic, a whole series of test apparatus was set up. They each involved tilting or reacting to changing visual input, or both. The test that I remember as being the most challenging, and the most bizarre, was when I was buckled into something like a parachute harness and placed in a vertical box. I was to keep standing as straight as I could while the scenery inside the box revolved and the floor I was standing on tilted in different directions. All I have to say is that it was good I was strapped in that harness! It kept me from falling, which I would have definitely done otherwise. I certainly could have passed for an inebriated man who was failing a sobriety test!

One thing I found in this testing was *exhaustion*! With the lost skills I had experienced from the head injury, when I struggled to maintain balance and coordination under challenge, I was straining to marshal forces that I was deficient in. Some patients may no longer possess the faculties to really hold up under these challenges. That does not mean they shouldn't fight the best they can. Personally, I *did* fight for it. I don't give up easily. In each one of those tests, I fought with whatever remnants I had left. When a patient is struggling in an area of some weakness, compensatory fighting is necessary, but it has its cost. I can appreciate the fact that test results on equipment like that are dependent on the residual ability of the patient. I realize also, though, that the results are conditional upon the struggle the patient is willing to wage! I suspect that those who interpret the tests must be willing to add a judgement factor to the results. Sometimes I wonder about other patients who don't fight as much! Do they end up on medicine they do not need or do some even end up on disability benefits?

Along the way of my journey for answers, I elected to get an opinion from a leading teaching institution in the state. I went for several visits to one of their staff neurologists in the appropriate clinic area. On my first visit, I sat in the reception room filling out a long, really long, questionnaire. I felt encouraged. I saw words and phrases that seemed to coincide with my dysfunction. I thought, they "get this!" I highlighted those for my wife as she sat next to me. I just knew I was going to get help! I went through that Dix-Hallpike test, this time wearing the fancy camera goggles, called Frenzel's glasses. It was somewhat reassuring that those experts found no more ready answers than were available in my home area. Unfortunately, despite the phraseology in the initial questionnaire, it did not seem that the doctor and I spoke the same language of dysfunction. When all was said and done, I got the distinct impression that my doctor there did not fully appreciate the depth of the difficulty I was fighting. That was the discouraging part.

My last extended testing was done by a behavioral psychologist, as I remember. I had pushed for this because I was still seeking explanations and validation. She spent several hours with me in all kinds of tests. She tested everything from my ability to recognize smells to timing me on placing puzzle pieces with my non-dominant hand. I never did figure out what all that meant. Dr. Blackburn just absorbed the results and kept on assisting me. Thank you, Doc!

Let me give you some modern hope in the way of resources that are available today. Such therapies were not available in years past, not even ten years ago. Two trends have come together to open the pocketbooks for researchers to investigate brain injury. Probably the first was the acknowledgement of chronic brain injury in some professional football players, an area of deep pockets. In addition, with the return of many of our soldiers who have suffered traumatic brain injury in theatre, both the government and some private institutions have intensified efforts to assess and treat victims of mild to severe brain injuries. Often, due to the setting of injury, it is difficult to distinguish between that which may be due to physical traumatic injury vs. the psychologic injury of Post-traumatic Stress Disorder (PTSD). Certainly, many soldiers suffer from the complexity of both. This can potentially lead to misdiagnosis and a less-than-the-best treatment plan. Unfortunately, many of these men and women returning from the war go from being aggressive warriors to being embarrassed, discouraged, and timid sufferers unwilling to fully admit to their issues. They still want to be perceived as tough soldiers and can be reluctant to confess how the symptoms are impacting their daily relationships and activities. Often, it is the household contact or loved one that must speak up. Unlike facing up to a visible war wound, these soldiers may not be wearing a purple heart and may not be respected for their sacrifice. They feel terribly exposed and may see their confession as weakness. Understanding and compassion from those surrounding the men and women who return can cause that door of isolation to crack open a bit. If love and support come through that door, help will follow.

As supporters and as sufferers, we have to be open to listen and talk to our tough-guy heroes. We must realize that they are trained to be stoic, not to be open. Reaching those who have been wounded in invisible ways takes time and caring. We also have to open our hearts to warriors who have suffered in training. Practicing for war is inherently dangerous. Many of our military victims can suffer traumatic brain injury without ever leaving for the area of battle. They are Americans who have chosen to serve to protect us. They must receive our full support, as well.

There are two therapies that are now available. I see them as developing areas that have already shown healing effect and are showing even greater future potential. One is Electronic Stimulation Therapy or

PrTMS- Personalized Repetitive Transcranial Magnetic Stimulation. The other is Cranial Electrotherapy using Alpha-Stim devices. These may be available in different areas. They appear to be worth a look and may be something you wish to bring up with your medical care provider.

SO, WHAT WAS IT REALLY LIKE? It was a discouraging and disheartening battle. Advanced testing and specialty care provided no additional fixes. Despite the investment of time, money, and hope, I never found a magic band-aid to heal my injury. But, I had to learn that basic lesson, and settle that false hope for a clinical miracle, before I could move on to the perspective of learning from my journey.

CHAPTER 11

The Universal Therapy

"Sometimes the questions are complicated and the answers are simple." Dr. Seuss

Let me address that worn out, run down, exhausted, out-of-gas feeling. It can come from many sources in your everyday life. It can come from the battles against mediocrity or the battle of the daily struggle against clean dishes, cooking, putting kids to bed, and balancing the checkbook. I certainly experienced exhaustion frequently during my clinical education and practice experience. Still, that kind of exhaustion is dependent on circumstances and recent loss of sleep. My condition was different after the head injury. No other time in my life have I experienced such pervasive, persistent exhaustion. My head demanded sleep.

First, it is well accepted that the greatest aid for brain healing is rest. Medicines have their place. Therapy is important. Support is essential. But, if you want your brain to heal, REST IT. This is especially true immediately after the injury! That means more sleep. That means quiet time. That means watching TV *or* reading, not watching TV *and* reading at the same time. It also means to actively plan to spend as much time as possible in low-stimulus environments. Avoid concerts and loudspeakers. Avoid blasts of bright light. Avoid unstable or rocking surfaces. Try to make it as easy on your brain as possible when you are not involved in necessary activity. Some of that necessary activity may be directed by your healthcare team as attempts are made to retrain your brain. Do your therapy, and then rest that brain.

While rest augments recovery during the first few weeks of acute injury, that is not the only time to utilize that bit of therapy. In my life and yours, there are times when we just have to perform at a high level, whether we feel like it or not. That above-and-beyond effort at concentration, multi-tasking, or exposure to noxious surroundings will take its toll. In the aftermath, rest is the best answer for recovery.

When I was a teenager, I could sleep the day away. That changed dramatically when I began training to be a physician. Sleep was often an entity that I got behind on. It would always make me feel bad in the pit of my stomach when I was truly sleep-deprived. I know what it is like to work the day, work all night without sleep, and then to work the next day. It is quite a task to maintain cheerfulness, not be grumpy, and also maintain mental sharpness. Functioning through sleep deprivation isn't fun any of the time, but it can be, and was for me, a learned skill. Under normal clinical demand, it was sometimes tough, but I was trained and conditioned to handle it. It was a matter of discipline, dedication, mental toughness, and commitment. Whenever I was behind on sleep, I would take advantage of the first chance I encountered to catch up.

That tough endurance component, that I had worked so many years to hone, was really put to a test after my injury. Between the condition and the medicines to help control the symptoms, I gave out of energy much earlier. You can expect that if you are having frequent dysfunction, as in headaches, spinning, imbalance, etc., you are going to have to expend more energy on anything you do. Whether it is driving, walking, reading, or doing the dishes, it will all take more of your concentration to focus and, thus, take more of your energy reserve. I might add that it may also affect your level of patience with yourself and others! It makes sense that if you burn more mental calories with increased effort at focus and concentration, you will wear out sooner. That is just simply the truth of biologic math! Think of this self-test: how long can you keep your eyelids scrunched down while you stare at an inanimate object, such as a doorknob? You will grow tired much more quickly than if you were just scanning around the room. Any intense concentration of focus is much more tiring. When you are fighting your dizziness or data-overload symptoms, you will be concentrating, and you will be tiring. My advice? Rest. And then rest some more!

I did go to a Certified Balance Therapist. She worked out of Dr. Maitland's office. She had Dr. Maitland's endorsement and direction; thus, I was on-board. I have discovered that the American Institute of Balance will certify physical therapists, occupational therapists, and audiologists, amongst other providers, after they take a prescribed course and get some experience. There may be other certifications that I am not aware of.

Under the guidance and instruction of the therapist, I spent a time going through a series of exercises. As I remember, part of that therapy involved trying to maintain balance on soft, couch-cushion-type surfaces. Some of that therapy had me balancing on cushions while purposely tilting, etc. I must admit I did not stick to those exercises for a long period of time. They tended to provoke my symptoms. I am sure that provocation was designed to slowly build my tolerance, in a controlled way, over time. For some patients, the exercises might be very helpful. It did not seem to be working for me. Perhaps I was just impatient. Have I told you I have issues with patience? Anyway, I rationalized that since I was working so hard and stressing my functioning in such a demanding career field, amongst a mine field of balance challenges, I could not afford to take any more time away from the rest I knew I needed.

I have referred to seeking an opinion from a teaching hospital in my state. I was told by my doctor there that the best way to recovery was to not give in to the "spinning." I was told to keep running; the exercise would be good for me. I guess the theory here was, if I ignored my symptoms, they would just resolve and disappear. That same doctor started me on an antidepressant drug. She told me she was sure it would help. She expected me to be a new person a month later. Truthfully, however, I never felt I was depressed through all of this. Yes, I got angry; and yes, I experienced grief over losing the old me, but I never gave in or lost my will to fight! While I admit I had emotions, I never gave up. Depression would have almost been a declaration of acceptance of my new limitations and I wasn't ready for that then. In my mind I was thinking there must be some other hidden advantage to this drug and that must be why she wants me to take it. So I took it and looked for the predicted improvement.

I am pretty sure that this practitioner, who expected me to have dramatic improvement in a month, did not really accept the depth of my injury. In retrospect, since this was early in her practice, even though she was in a sub-specialty practice, my issues may have outweighed her experience. A limitation of therapeutic options and a one-size-fits-all treatment may reflect on the practitioner who does not really appreciate the condition he or she is charged with managing. I was struggling daily to "ignore the symptoms" and keep my life together. This approach had *not* worked. And that is why I was seeking help! Unfortunately, after that month on the antidepressant, I saw no change in anything. Over time, I did not stay with that medicine *or* with that doctor.

I should be fair. Maybe I was too sensitive to being diagnosed as depressed. Depression is a clinical state that may be chronic and last for years or it may be situational and be related to current events or problems. I may have had some component of depression, but I did not see it. I saw my struggles as anger and grief! Yes, I got angry over this! I was angry that I couldn't stay in charge of it all! That was a real loss for me. I didn't realize at the time that the anger was part of my battle against God's control in my life. That lesson was slow to sink in! I wanted to be the one in the driver's seat! Yes, I experienced grief over losing the old me and my capabilities. I literally mourned my independence and ability to perform athletically at a high level. While I admit I felt a real loss, I never gave up. I never gave in or lost my will to fight!

I have mentioned the fight within me numerous times. I come from what might be referred to as a humble background. I watched both my parents suffer and die from cancer. My dad had succumbed first. He had no life insurance. Mom became a seamstress at a clothing store, earning very little income. I saw her forced to sell our home and become dependent in government-subsidized housing. Then, I witnessed my mother's long struggle with cancer. Her fight ended right after I completed my medical school requirements. Both my parents were gone; they were much too young.

There was really no money in the bank for me. All during this time, I was doing what I could do. I was studying, looking for an educational way out of this situation. I was working part-time, when feasible. There was even one stretch in college when I was working and balancing three part-time jobs at once. As I watched both my parents struggle and die from disease, I realized I would be on my own. It was up to me to build a future and a life of success. With the help of God, I would build into that future. The past helped to make me; perhaps it filled me with understanding and compassion, and it taught me to be tough. But I would not dwell in the past. I would not make excuses or compromise because I had been dealt some difficult cards. Little did I know of the burdensome cards of head injury still in the deck. I would take events as they came and do my best to keep an eye on the future by overcoming any present challenges! Life has to be about looking forward to tomorrow, not looking back at yesterday. We are to follow the light of our calling. We can only follow as we keep our heads up and our eyes focused into the future. You will never make it out of the spiritual desert if you have your head down, watching your feet. In order to make progressive steps, you must fixate on your goal on the opposite side of the challenge. As denoted by the apostle Paul in Philippians 3:13-14, "...Forgetting what is behind and straining toward what is ahead, I press on toward the goal to win the prize for which God has called me heavenward in Christ Jesus."

I have been a runner for a long time. It was a way for me to wind down from the day's stress and to increase my fitness. I remember the joy of taking my running shoes with me if I went on a trip. Setting out to investigate, running step by step, is really a great way to see new surroundings and experience the community. When home, I often ran at the end of the day, to burn off stress and frustration, before supper and family time. A great guy, a YMCA director, and a good friend of mine, Rick Callebs, got me into marathoning. Over time, I ran all the lengths up to and including marathon, running a total of eleven marathons during that time in my life. You have read that my Tybee concussion coincided with plans to run a half-marathon the following day. As I told you, that did not work out. I was also committed to running a half-marathon with another young man and good guy, Rex Brooking. He lives in the Cincinnati area and we were to run the half-marathon at the annual Flying Pig Marathon running event there! I had participated in that event before and had run the full marathon. This was to be a little more relaxed!

Well, have you ever discovered that when you plan trips or activities, you do so full of anticipation and excitement? As time draws closer to your commitment, circumstances may develop to complicate your availability or your interest. Seems to work that way for me! Well, my interest was still strong. I wanted to see Rex and the guys, and I wanted to have all the usual fun. My ability was still there, such as it was. It was more like I was having an internal-equipment malfunction! The Pig is run in early May. That would have been about 3 months after my concussion. I was doing as I was told and continuing to run. It was hard. That "spacey" sensation was a common companion following me on my runs. I would sometimes have to struggle with balance and sometimes struggle with disorientation. Staggering was an occasional challenge.

I well remember that Pig half-marathon. It was a fight all the way. Rex is this athletically built, tall and fit, younger version of what I never was! He is a true runner. I wanted to help him, not hinder him. I wanted to keep up a pace that we could both enjoy and sustain over the thirteen-plus miles. That was a tough order. I could tell that the running was affecting my perceptions and disrupting my spatial orientation. In addition to my balance issues, something I had eaten the day before was not agreeing with me. That would cause a delay somewhere along the way. Rex was never fully aware of how I was struggling, but I am sure I burned more calories per mile than I would have months before. He ended up being my beacon who kept me on a straight course. As I struggled, I encouraged him to go ahead. He elected to stay with me. I told you; he is a good guy! We finished in a good time: a little under two hours, I believe. We could be proud of our accomplishment, but I could embrace that feeling of success only after I sat and recovered!

When I review information sources now, I see comments all over the place about the benefit of exercise while experiencing a post-concussion effect. One extreme is to just keep going. This assumes that the jogging won't hurt and that it will lead you back to your normal life sooner. A more middle-of-the-road policy is to encourage exercise, but to back off before you get to the level of provoking your symptoms. Exercise is good for our cardiovascular health and it can be very empowering to do "something" to help yourself during this challenging time. Theoretically, if you avoid symptoms, you also avoid aggravation of your healing tissues. At the other extreme, some do recommend avoiding impactful exercise until your symptoms have significantly resolved. You will have to take your physician's advice, based on your condition. You also need to use your common sense a little more than I did. My opinion is that provoking symptoms must be limited and controlled for expeditious healing to occur. For me, I should have limited my running more. Frankly though, I think if I had only run to the point of symptoms, I would not have run at all!

My take on all this is partially based on my reading, but it is based more on my experience. Most concussions that do not involve severe head trauma may not show up on a typical MRI. That is because the injury is on the cellular level, a level not visible on an MRI scan. Neurons, or nerve cells, are highly complex entities. Each nerve cell has multiple communications with other cells. In fact, to study this connectivity, and the breadth of how nerve cells communicate, is to discover the miraculous! Concussion is described as: the brain, surrounded by its cerebrospinal fluid, sloshing back and forth with severe enough impact to provoke injury. As I described earlier in relation to my theoretical sites of injury, it is very understandable how such injury, such acceleration and deceleration in a soft organ, could disrupt or tear many of these connections that are so small they are invisible to the naked eye. Once the cellular disruptions occur, the difficulty of brain communication is increased. For a parallel comparison, think of a bridge that is washed out. You won't be able to cross the river in that area. You will have to learn a detour to get to the same eventual destination. It may take time to find and accomplish that detour. You will eventually end up at the same goal, but the journey will be more difficult and time-consuming, and you will burn more gas. The brain reacts in much the same way. When a primary path is disrupted, the healing mechanism involves developing new flow patterns around the site of loss. While this detouring is being formed, we encounter dysfunction of our usual faculties. This level of injury, cellular tearing, is well below the view of an MRI. It would require putting a microscope in your head somehow to find these torn communicators.

I know that neurologic healing is slow, and I know it takes longer as we get older. There also is variation in the expanse of the injury each of us receives and a variation in how each of us heals such sensitive and important tissue. I erred in following the aggressive direction of freedom I was given. Realize, I was a runner. It was part of who I was. I wanted to keep running and when they told me it would be good for me, I bolted on a run! Unfortunately, my common sense was yelling, "YOU KNOW

BETTER!" By the way, it was not just *my* common sense. My wife, Mary's, common sense was active, as well. She was worried that I was inhibiting healing and perhaps causing more damage. I am fortunate that I did not stumble, fall, and cause further setback with another head injury! I could tell, though, as I ran, that I was aggravating my symptoms. I finished that half-marathon in Ohio. It wasn't easy. In retrospect, it wasn't smart, and it wasn't how I should have cared for myself. I remember feeling totally spacey. I remember staggering. I remember the sides of the course looking strange. And I remember being miserable afterwards from pressure, sitting up against a wall with my body stopped and still but my brain continuing to move. The movement still going on in my head forced me to sit against a fixed surface and wait for my brain to relax and calm down enough for me to be fully interactive with my friends. I had "spaced" out.

By the way, as I went through my medical training, I was instructed to never accept the term "dizzy" from a patient. I was taught that the term was non-specific and not helpful. I was trained to ask, "What do you mean by dizzy?" In a way, that was good training. As I have noted before, it can be just about impossible to label your symptoms in a way that others will know what you mean. One man's dizzy may be something different to the other ten people that are also using that term. It is very appropriate for me as a clinician to try and understand what you are feeling. I need to ask, "What do you mean by that?" It is also very appropriate that you, as the patient, try to give the physician as much information about your distress as possible. Try not to use one-word labels that may mean different things to different people. You may even want to try and practice your description before you go to the doctor. When the doctor asks you a pointed question, trying to come up with a quick response about a strange feeling can be difficult anytime. It is especially difficult during a time of cognitive dysfunction.

To this point in my writing here, I *have* limited my use of that term "dizzy." Yet, when I think about it, "dizzy" is as good a term as "spinning" or "pressure." No one word will describe your dysfunction. Try to use succinct sentences in a short paragraph to inform your physician. Both you and the physician trying to help you may benefit from some prepared thoughts. As for me, when we would travel to the doctor's office, my wife would quiz me with, "What are you going to tell the doctor?" If my answers excluded some detail she thought was significant, she would point that out to me. It was helpful to review how I had been doing and be prepared to give more than a quick, short answer to questions. There was nothing more important than working with my medical-care-support team to improve my management.

If this book serves its purpose, you may see some of your struggles in my wording. Sharing some of these terms or concepts with your doctor may be a way to open a discussion.

SO, WHAT WAS IT REALLY LIKE? It was discouraging. I was tempted to feel defeated, but I would not give up. I failed in the art of common sense. Compromise and prudence were lessons I did not easily learn!

CHAPTER 12

Lessons of the First Decade

"Don't let what you can't do, stop you from doing what you can do." John Wooden

"If you choose to magnify what you have lost, you are going to live in what you have lost." Steven Furtick

I have often reflected on how a moment in time can impact a lifetime. I have seen it so often. In a negative way, a car crash can lead to death or disability. In a positive way, the moment of birth is always a life-changer! In my life, I have been blessed all along the way. My road has been downhill and smooth, as I see it. There was that day in 2004 that forced a fork in the road. I stumbled and stuttered but eventually chose the right path around that boulder that was dropped in my stream of planning. It hasn't been easy, and it certainly has not occurred without help from many sources. But my downstream life is a pleasant one. I have grown to a point that I can now be thankful for the challenges that have forced the changes.

I have learned so much through this odyssey of injury. Sharing my gains may help you in your struggles. My first lesson was a bitter one. I was not the same hyper-functional person and professional I had always previously been. I could not be as active or involved in the community. I had to cut down on my hours of activity. I could not be as adventuresome hiking by myself or running in new areas. My playing field had shrunk!

The scriptures tell us in Romans 8:28, "And we know that in all things God works for the good of those who love Him, who have been called according to His purpose." Back during those first few years, I was not ready for that lesson. In fact, I was feeling grief over my lost independence and capabilities. It was as if part of my self-image had died! It was as if I was looking in a broken mirror and part of that glass with its mirror-image was missing! I could no longer, as the song says, "climb every mountain." It seemed as though I was down to stumbling over mole hills and needing help, sometimes, to even do that. My feeling of loss lasted a long time. For me, in some limited ways, this resembled losing a loved one, someone whom you have shared a home with, for instance. Not only do you experience the shock of loss and the empty chair at the table, you also continue to encounter items that remind you of your loved one for a long time to come. Each day, I was confronted by my *can'ts*, *couldn'ts*, and *wouldn'ts*, and that took me a long time to get past. Mary was ever the loving wife, and she accepted the new me, the new normal, well ahead of the time that I could come to terms with the reality of my limitations.

Somewhere along this way of grief and loss I had a friend come to visit me. She was from our church. She and my wife have spent more time together over the years, and I was just peripheral to that relationship. Because of their closeness, she was one of the few people somewhat clued-in to the depth of my problem. When she called and asked to come see me, I accepted. We sat around the table. She told me that she felt led by God to come visit with me. She believed He had given her a message for my ear and my spirit. That message was this: I needed to look upon the head injury as a blessing; that I would actually be better off because of it! WOW! I was not anywhere near ready for that message. I did not deny her earnestness or her meaning; I just was not ready to accept it. It would be well into that first decade before I could acknowledge such. And that was really through adapting and healing over time, both physically and spiritually. Her message continued to echo within me until I could grow and accept it. Time allowed me such a perspective.

I have noted that I live in a small town. I always felt that part of my mission was to see, as I would say, beyond the exam table into the community. Over the years prior to my injury, in addition to a busy practice, I was prominent in civic and hospital positions. I did things that doctors do not often feel led to do. In the hospital, I served obligatory posts like being chairman of the Ob/Gyn Department. I also served two terms as Chief of Staff. In the community, I held down several offices. I spent time as an elected officer in the Chamber of Commerce and completed a term as president. I was in the Kiwanis Club for a while, leading committees and serving as an officer there. My path with Kiwanis eventually parted, and later I became active in the Rotary Club, serving as my club's president and then going on to serve as an assistant district governor. Yes, I was busy and involved: pursuing many different avenues, and assuming responsibilities where I thought my talents might serve the common purpose.

In a way, that all changed for the better after my injury. I have never stopped helping my community when I can. I just feel that doctors are typically some of the most highly compensated and capable individuals in any small town. We physicians have each been blessed, and we owe our current success to the community. My view is that we, as physicians, serve the communities in helping to maintain wellness, treat disease, and encourage healthy lifestyles. That is a great service. When possible, we can serve in other ways that are in addition to our professional hours. And we can work to better our communities in more ways than just healthcare.

The new me could not flash around like the old me. I could not keep going to evening meetings, rush out at lunch, or tie up my Saturdays. It was time to walk a path closer to my Christian calling. Prior to settling in Bainbridge as the place we would call home, I was not a particularly devoted follower. Sure, we went to church; but I was, more than anything else, someone holding down a pew. My wife has always been the spiritual one. She was raised in the home of a man who answered a mid-life calling to become a Methodist minister and she was "always in the church." Unlike some preachers' kids, she thrived there, and her spiritual side is very prominent.

I remember, as my time in the USAF was drawing to a close, I was looking for a place to go into private practice. I was considering multiple opportunities. One of those opportunities was Bainbridge. I remember the day I drove into Bainbridge for my interview. It was the first potential site that I visited, to consider if this community and hospital could possibly be our future home. As we drove down the main thoroughfare in town, Shotwell Street, before I even stopped to talk with anyone, God sat on my heart and said something to the effect of, "This is where I want you." I am as sure of that as I am of anything. At that instant, I *knew* that Bainbridge was where I belonged. The inner conviction impressed me to such an extent that I cancelled future interviews. I didn't decide because of the hospital facilities or the number of patients or the average income in the area. Those might have even been negatives. I did not even feel the need to ask a lot of questions. This major choice was made because I decided to be obedient to His guidance. Without a doubt, I felt utterly compelled and confident that we were to settle in Bainbridge.

We joined the United Methodist Church and I became active in teaching and sharing. That was something I had never done before. Years later, as I was coming to terms with the limitations posed by my head condition, my activities outside my practice became more restricted and more church centered. I have gone on to lead men's groups, teach Sunday School and Bible studies, and have been known to preach occasionally. God set the table for all that and perhaps He slowed me down in order for me to adapt more to His plan!

There are also practical things I have learned. Bending over can cause me to spin. So, what do I need to do? I need to limit bending down. Every hardware and utility store carries implements that allow you to pick things up off the ground, whether it be pinecones and sticks outside, or dropped objects inside. That has made a difference for me. If I need to tend to something on the floor, I will most often just sit down right on the floor to maintain that ol' even keel and limit inverting my head.

If there is an item that I need to put up, but use frequently, it needs to go onto a shelf or in a drawer that does not cause me to bend. Simple, but profound. Limiting aberrant extremes keeps me more functional. Limiting climbing on stools and ladders is also wise!

Have I mentioned, "I am not patient"? Yes, I have, several times. That is because it is so true. However, this injury challenge has taught me more in the way of tolerance and patience than I have ever known before. I used to be the ramrod. If we were going on vacation, I was pushing and demanding, "Let's go!" I cannot do that anymore. I am too dependent on cooperation of others for me to be bossy. My wife has been doing all of the driving of any length or complexity. Shall we say, she is not the aggressive driver I always was! Even as a rider, I have mellowed. I have gone from, "You know you have plenty of room to pass," to internalizing the belief that there is just not often a reason to hurry to such an extent. The raging beast has calmed!

Memory is relative. My memory function is fine now, at least I think so. What I think, or you think about your own memory, is really the most critical way to assess that function. Some people may say, "You can't remember anything." I know better. In areas where I need to remember accurately, I have that peripheral memory of paper and pen in my pocket, and I get by.

The truth hurts sometimes. It hurts the recipient *and* the bearer, perhaps. I may not remember what you said or what you planned because it just was not significant or important to me at the time I heard it. "Sorry," I guess. Guys, especially, know this is true. By the way, when someone says, "Don't you remember, I told you?", and you do not remember the conversation, who is really at fault? Is it *your* memory or *their* memory that is incorrect? I leave you with that recurring question. For me, I choose to not always bear the burden of claiming to be the one with the incorrect, failed memory. Suffice it to say, I do not let remembering less than 100 percent of daily non-clinical details burden me.

I am not as capable as I was once was, but that does not mean I am incapable. I am not as able as I once was, but that does not mean I am disabled! I have had a lot of time to make adjustments now. Give me time and I can get whatever done, at least as well as I have always been able to. I can generally manage a way around to limit my head stressors. I just have to plan and allow more flexibility sometimes.

I am more dependent than ever, but that is alright! What I have lost in independence, I have gained in relationship. My daughter, Laura, because she lived at home part of this time, has seen me more vulnerable than I would have desired. She was one of the ones who would come out and lead me from my truck into the house at the end of the day. She saw me, her tough-guy dad, filled to tears with emotions in the early days. She and my wife have seen me at my weakest, but that is okay, as well. I am no longer as domineering as I once was. In fact, I sometimes approach being a "real pussycat." Being more available, more vulnerable, more patient, and more interactive has led to better multi-faceted, in-depth relationships.

Not being the dominant driver is okay! You know you can appreciate the scenery along the road much better if you are not driving. When my head will not allow such, I look down and get in reading time. It is safer for me to be dysfunctional in the passenger's seat! When my head will allow, I can look out the windows and see vistas that I never really noticed before. Smelling the roses along the way, "ain't all bad." Slowing down can be good!

There are always forks in the road. If you are fortunate, you may be allowed to decide which path to follow. After my fall, if I had continued to follow the path of denial and had not sought out assistance, my failures would eventually have become obvious, affecting my practice and my family. After much early frustration and failure to maintain the status quo, I chose the path to reach out for help. My family has been incredibly supportive. My office team was there for me! My professional medical assistance, from all sources, has provided continuing understanding and guidance. I am in a better place because I chose to be vulnerable within a circle of support, one I knew I could trust.

SO, WHAT WAS IT REALLY LIKE? I experienced self-questioning, at a time when I thought I had my life together. I had my family, my career, and "my" plan for life! Now, all that seemed to be in doubt. I wasn't sure if there was a threat to my financially providing for my family. I wasn't sure that I would be able to continue to answer the bell for my practice. I most assuredly did not understand what might happen with my memory and my thinking talents over time.

This forced me to redefine myself. I had always been in the driver's seat. I determined my path. I acknowledged God, but I did not often wait for His direction. While my wife may have been driving the car, my faith was now teaching me that God was to be in the driver's seat in my life! I was to be along for the ride to see what He had in mind for me. My life had never really been about being in the passenger seat, literally or figuratively! Suddenly, I found myself being forced to reassess all that. Whereas, before the injury, I was always the boss in my planning and in my family, now there are many times that I am literally forced to follow. Having to be "along for the ride" has given me a new perspective. In fact, this new perspective is reflected in many areas of my life. This has led to my becoming more dependent on His guidance in my life. That *patience* thing has evolved. Not being in the lead has allowed me a different perspective and more time for reflection. Smelling the flowers along the way has gained in value. My definition of myself was indeed altered, but in an incredibly positive, accepting, and loving way! For that, I am thankful.

While the nurses I worked with in the office and in the hospital knew things had changed, they never really were let in on the full extent of my problems. Do not deny what you cannot hide. That does not mean you need to sit everybody down for a dissertation on your disability. Like when your kid asks, "Where do babies come from?", tell them what they need to know and can understand at the time. The child, or the nurse in my case, is not really asking for a total explanation. They want an answer for what they have seen or what they have contemplated. Often for me, it was just a matter of saying, "I need to sit here a few minutes," and that was enough.

Not everyone is understanding! While it is essential to be honest with those closest to you, there are some who will not understand. To make off-handed remarks such as, "That is just my head acting up," most likely will not be understood and perhaps will cause ridicule. Vulnerability within the *incorrect* setting may lead to loss of confidence towards you and loss of community with others. Be careful how and when you open yourself up. I would even recommend that you be careful how you phrase some of your challenges when you first meet a medical professional that you have sought out to help you. Start with the basics; add more details as time and confidence grow.

I must make note of another scripture here. Proverbs, the 31st chapter, addresses the gift of a good wife. My favorite verses are 10 and 12: "A wife of noble character who can find? She is worth far more than rubies. She brings him good, not harm, all the days of her life." My relationship with my wife has deepened over time, as it should. Unfortunately, many find that the developments of life interfere with that relational maturation. You may face one of those forks in the road which forces a decision: do you push away, or do you pull closer? My wife saw the look in my eyes the day after my fall on Tybee. From that point forward she put her self-interest to the side to provide for me, to tend to my new needs, and to try to help me understand what was happening. She took over the driving without complaint or belittling me. She was often the voice of caution when I was moving in ways we both knew were not in my best interest. She tolerated my responses when I was not always thankful for such limiting guidance. She helped me plan appointments with doctors or therapy and coordinated it with my office schedule. She helped me get to work if I needed it, and she basically poured herself out as an offering for my well-being. We have built a marriage and a family. Along the way, through our plenty and through our pain, we have grown closer and have continued to build relationship. In fact, we have probably done more building since my injury. I give her and God, the Inventor of love, all the credit.

CHAPTER 13

Honesty

"He who guards his mouth and his tongue keeps himself from calamity." Proverbs 21:23

I just could not write this book without an emphasis on communication and honesty. Openness and honesty are essential and yet must be guarded during your recovery. Let me touch on how I have seen this.

According to Danielle Van Alst, a psychologist, author, and counselor, there are acceptable reasons to be guarded. She says, "Being a completely open book with everyone who shows you a little attention can cause a lot of unnecessary drama. Use your judgement and be discerning of who you let in and you can save yourself a whole lot of headaches. Sometimes, you have to be guarded. It's just necessary."

Honesty was very difficult for me at first. Before I could consider how I would communicate the new me to others, I first had to deal with my own realization. As I have mentioned, I was in denial. I was not willing to be honest with myself. I denied the extent of the injury, the limitations it was imposing, and the considerations of the future implications. By assuming that tomorrow would be better and that I did not really have a problem, I led myself to put off appropriate medical intervention. It is true that there was no immediate intervention that *would* heal the injury of concussion or mild traumatic brain injury. However, that does not mean that evaluation, timely advice, and intervention would not have been of benefit to me. The fact that I was struggling and only sought professional assistance after an orthopedist made me go is evidence enough of my denial.

Did I worry Mary needlessly during this time? Most probably. Did I do something inadvisable that I should not have done? Again, most probably. Did my pig-headed obstinance force a further disruption of my brain or limit its healing, because I failed to become more conservative in my activities sooner? I do not have answers for that question. Maybe I just do not want to confess my reluctance to "wake up and smell the coffee." I do have a feeling, as I look back, that my failure to slow down sooner caused my symptoms to worsen and drag on. Because slowing down and limiting impacts might have led to less disruption in my life for years thereafter, I wish I would have been honest with myself sooner.

I hope that you are fortunate enough to have a life partner, sibling, or friend who will support you, no matter what. My wife has proven herself to be just such a caring and giving person. I give her the earthly credit for keeping me headed in helpful directions. I was not honest with Mary at first. She had to see my eyes fixating and guess what was happening. True, I wasn't sure myself early on. However, looking back, I know that I hid from her my own concerns over what all these symptoms could mean. After all, I am a medical professional. While head injuries were not primary to my practice, I have encountered enough patients along the way to know that my condition could be very serious with multifaceted implications. At home, I owed Mary better. I should have reached out with my situational analysis much sooner and more openly to the one I was closest to. I ask you, when your thinking is not clear, is that not when you need the most counsel? I should have been more completely honest with my wife! I encourage you to do better than I did.

My beautiful daughter, Laura, was exposed to my dysfunctions. She asked very few questions; she just loved me. My strong son, Tal, who was on his own and out of state, was mainly clued in by his sister and remained supportive and understanding. I am sure that much in this book will be a surprise to him. As for my brother, brothers-in-law, sisters-in-law, and other extended family, distance and discretion ruled the day. They may have their concepts altered and stretched through this book, as well. I was comforted, knowing that they cared about me and whatever was going on.

One thing I did not drag my feet on was watching out for my patients. I had to ensure safety for each of them. My actions reveal that this was a very early priority. I was wanting to guarantee that my thought processes were active and correct in the clinical setting. It is evident that I was being very careful, thinking clearly enough to set up safety nets in my practice. I discussed patient care with my partner, I asked my office assistant to react if she saw me behave in any concerning way, and I apprised the nurses in Labor and Delivery, as well as the Operating Room, in appropriate ways.

I have told you how important it is to have a nucleus of individuals in your life during your recovery. This cannot be over-emphasized. However, those who are the support persons to you may not all need to know the whole story. In fact, trying to explain everything you are feeling, and everything that is changing in your perceptions, will probably go way overboard as to what your support team cares to know. Announcing a treatise concerning the extent of your injury, your medical interventions, and any medicines you have begun, is not indicated and may be distracting or confusing. For instance, I have mentioned Kathy Johnson. She was a wonderful office assistant for many years. She was charged with conducting patients through their clinical visit and assisting me in all ways possible. She did not really need to know about my CT scans, the theory of Vestibular Migraines, or how much trouble I had just getting home every day. She did know I had suffered a concussion, I needed to rest at lunch, and that sometimes I was moving slower than usual. These were things she could help me to manage. As my wife had learned, Kathy would watch my eyes. She would know when I was struggling more significantly. It was enough for her to know that I was "dizzy" and that I needed time.

Even my partner at the time, the one who would have to cover for me, Dr. Dean Burke, was never really treated to a treatise on my evaluation and current symptoms. It was enough for me to reach out and tell him what I needed. We had been together long enough at that point in our practice to have sown a crop of confidence and trust. I am very grateful that he was so willing to stay close during this time. The nurses I worked with were aware that I had issues, especially with those movements of the operating table I mentioned. It was enough for them to know that I was having some balance issues and that I had to be careful, in new ways!

I never chose to be deceptive. I did not lie. I answered questions as they were posed. But I *did* follow lawyer rules: I would answer the question and only the question. Any question posed to me directly deserved a direct answer. I assumed the query was not offered, and it was not received, as an open invitation to "explain it all." Fortunately, the questions I received usually came from loving, concerned friends and nurse colleagues. I felt their caring, and that is always good.

The city that I live in is a town of less than 13,000, in a county of around 25,000 people. We also attracted patients from surrounding areas. I had practiced in this area for seventeen years at the time of my injury. As previously shared, I had also been very active in the community with church, the Chamber of Commerce, civic clubs, and charities. I was known for my amateur photography and was fairly frequently called upon to give talks to local groups. In addition, I wrote medical articles for the local newspaper, *The Post-Searchlight*. All of this led to my being very recognizable in the community. I always joked that in a small town where everybody knows who you are, you have to watch your behavior in public. Fighting with a spouse, being inebriated, or other types of scenes would get around faster than blue dye in a glass of water. Being composed and under control is not a bad thing. And it is especially expected of someone who may deliver your daughter's baby, etc. That public image was one that I had worked hard to earn. It did not affect my image for someone to see my wife driving me around. That was an okay compromise. It *would* have affected my image if I had had a wreck or if I had walked unsteadily down the street like I was drunk. My time in the public was curtailed and was usually limited by my being accompanied by my wife. I knew that I was taking the precautions necessary to render safe medical care. I also knew that, with the rumor mill of a small town, it would have been very destructive to have the rumor spread that I was "brain damaged." Rumors do not specify details accurately and certainly are not generally spread in a positive or helpful manner. We did not publicize my condition. It would have done no public or private good to bring unneeded questioning to the thoughts of patients in the community. I was being very objective. I was seeking counsel from my physician and my partner. There was no doubt in my mind that I was still needed and useful in our small town that was chronically short of medical doctors. I had to keep functioning to the full extent possible, with safety ever present in my plan.

Honesty with your medical professionals is essential. There is no way around that. Your doctor cannot adequately prescribe a therapeutic plan if he/she does not know the extent of your problems. This is especially true with post-concussion syndrome and mild traumatic brain injury. The usual yardsticks that medical professionals use to assess injury, like CT scans and MRIs, do not show the extent of your injury. You, as the one who is experiencing the chaos of your brain function, have to be open, descriptive, and informative as to how you are impacted. Your healthcare provider needs to know how you usually function in your home and your job and how that has been altered by your current symptoms.

Remember though, I have already suggested that you may want to hold back on some of your more bizarre perceptual challenges until the basics have been set. When I mentioned the sort of hallucinations I experienced early-on (perceiving mailboxes as people) to one of the physicians I encountered, I got a very strange look! I am pretty sure that at that point, she was at least considering if I needed to be seen in the psychiatric clinic instead of the neurology clinic!

In your initial assessments after a head injury, there is so much to accomplish. Tests have to be ordered and interpreted; plans have to be formed. There will be opportunity down the road to develop, and more fully share, the nuances of what you are encountering. Start with the basics: what, when, and how. Progress to the symptoms that are causing you the most day-to-day challenges. Answer any questions fully and honestly. As time goes by, truthfully fill out the details of your problems or issues. Be honest, as well, during follow-up visits when the doctor asks you how you are doing. Your physician should be most motivated by a desire to help you survive in the mainstream of life. They seriously want to know if whatever therapy you have embarked upon is really helping. Today's medical practitioner has many medicines and other types of therapy, as well as cogent advice. If what you are trying is not adequately controlling your issues, do not be stubbornly stoic. Speak up honestly; there may be a better alternative.

There is one final aspect to this honesty issue that I want to especially address. When I did begin to realize the reality of my injury, the limitations of my condition, and the unknown of tomorrow, I was concerned. I practiced in this small town where I had to control potentially critical health issues in a clear and definitive fashion. Similar potential risk could be true of anyone who has to do high-voltage wiring or operate a large table saw, etc. First, for your sake and the sake of others, you have to be safe and in control. Well, that was my primary concern from the first day I recognized problems with my surroundings. I may not have grasped anything about the potential for long-term issues then, but it did not really matter at that point. My primary focus had to be safety from the first day back in the office. In my case, as I mentioned, I immediately set up those safety nets, bringing in my practice partner and seeking outside assurances from those who were professionally evaluating me.

As I traveled the road of my journey, I became concerned that I might not be able to maintain the highest level of function, that there was the potential that the medicine I was given might not hold me, or that my condition might worsen. After all, when we are confronted with what we think are memory issues, don't we all consider, "Could this be the first stages of Alzheimer's disease?" I even reached out to one of the doctors and asked, "What if I can't continue to do my job?" Fortunately, I never felt I had to pursue that issue further. That will not always be the case. Depending on your injury and your occupation, you may find yourself over that line. When is it time to say, "I can't continue to do this"? Once you have made that statement, you may end up being dependent on the opinions of medical professionals, the adjusters of your disability insurance, or the bureaucrats of the Social Security Administration. So, before you make that statement, include your medical professional in the discussion, as you carefully process your issues. If, honestly, you are in a situation that can be hazardous for you or others, that medical professional will be your ally. Be open and honest!

SO, WHAT WAS IT REALLY LIKE? The tough part was admitting to myself that my world had changed and that it was going to persist. That was *very* tough. On the basis of devotion to my wife, opening up to her was a natural next step. Through the years in my community and through my practice, I had built a reputation for integrity and being trustworthy. With that basis, I was surrounded by supporters; my "weakness" became an opportunity to learn about love. For our soldiers and other warriors, who are suffering through wounds and alterations, support is out there for you, as well.

CHAPTER 14

The Caregiver's Perspective, Introduction to Mary's Experience

"Life is about change. Sometimes it is painful. Sometimes it is beautiful. But most of the time, it's both." Lana Lang

You, as readers of this odyssey, have only heard my side. There is so much to the story and it has so many angles. I have talked about support from those around me. The love and loyalty tendered to me was very gracious. Thankful is an understatement from me, in my attempt to address those who hung in there and helped me progress from where I was, to where I needed to be. I am sure that Kathy, at the office, could relate observations and opinions. Still, she only saw one aspect of my functioning. She only saw me in the office setting. I am sure an operating-room nurse or two could remember some bizarre angles to my story, as well.

None of those surrounding me, and none of those in my inner circle, saw my struggles as clearly as did my wife. Mary has been committed to our marriage since before the ceremony. She has been loving and loyal through medical school and residency: times when I surely could not have been much fun! She took care of our children and accepted my being away at the hospital during Thanksgivings, Christmases, birthdays, and anniversaries. She knew my calling. And she, somehow, rose above those disappointments.

I have told you about the long hours of residency. Well, during that time, we were raising our son, Tal. I give my wife all the credit for his integrity and sound footing. She was there for him.

In some ways though, I believe residency was training for her, also. I was in training for the doctor lifestyle and the assumption of heavy responsibility. She was being trained in independence and the assumption of heavy responsibility at home. She was raised by a father who was a fix-it man. I helped show her a few things, and she took off from there. She doesn't like electricity things, but she is all over plumbing! She handled the food, the budget, the house, the bills, and the children. She made decisions on her own and she accomplished her efforts with a child or two always in her charge. She has been a grandly successful mother and wife.

Mary took our marriage vows seriously. There was never a question in her mind if she could live with the "visitor from a foreign planet" that I had become. Through "sickness and health," she has been with me, strongly at my side. To be honest, she has not always just been at my side. During those times of struggle, she often took the lead. Yes, she took on all the driving; but she did more than that. She sat with me when my "spinning" was bad; she let me sleep, when she would have had other plans; she was a sounding board for decision-making; and she was a counsel for direction or guidance. I owe so much to her. I know that you will benefit from her perspective.

CHAPTER 15

Mary's Experience

By the time Don and I moved to Bainbridge, we had already experienced a lot of life. After completing college, surviving medical school, enduring residency, and serving in the USAF for almost four years, we had a yen for a more settled life. Married, at this point, for eleven years, we had two young children, a need to put down some roots, and a great excitement for private practice in small-town Georgia.

We both became quite involved in church and civic activities. As the years clicked along, I was, of course, the principal one for helping out with any school activities. It was obvious from the get-go that the commitments and workload for an OB/GYN were going to require understanding and patience on my part and could potentially take a toll on our relationship. We safeguarded our family unit in every way we possibly could. I can honestly say I have never resented the sheer time commitment for Don's profession. And the reason is simple: he felt called, like divinely called, to his occupation. His sense of compassion, caring, and conviction for rendering superb medical care became his driving force.

Only those who are married to physicians really appreciate all that is required of them. In our case, the expectations for an obstetrician/gynecologist are quite daunting. There are full days in the office, stressful emergency issues with deliveries, up lots of nights, on-call seemingly constantly, much reading and studying to stay current on medical issues and to maintain Board certification; it's an all-consuming profession. But when you love what you do, and you feel that God has called you to it, you just accept the responsibilities and move forward. I worked very hard at helping our kids to be really tolerant of their Dad's demanding life.

So much about our family life was wonderful, and we were blessed. Healthy children, quiet neighborhood, special friends; you get the picture. What more could we want? Don was absolutely content in his work and never spoke of change or retirement. He stayed busy with club activities, church, etc., and he had settled into a bit of an exercise routine for staying fit and relieving stress.

Well, one thing led to another and before long he was an active, participating member of the local running club. Oak City Running Club to be exact. This small, but very enthusiastic, group of adults ran together regularly. They planned 5K runs and such, and often participated in events at Tallahassee and other tri-state locations nearby. I'm told that it's the endorphins within a person's brain, rushing or surging involuntarily as a response to exercising, that supposedly create a true sense of enjoyment. These folks had that, for sure: an enjoyment for running.

Then came the day when my husband announced that he was going to run a marathon. "You're doing what?!," I asked. I was stunned. That's a whole lot different from running a three-mile route in the neighborhood a few days a week. Despite my best arguments, nothing would persuade him to re-think that decision. So, at age forty, my level-headed husband embarked on yet another very time-consuming endeavor. Since I am the more practical of the two of us, I could find absolutely *no* redeeming or rewarding aspects to this new passion of his. He had already had several orthopedic injuries and surgeries. I was very concerned about the physical impact this would have on his knees, ankles, and hips. Then there was the "minor" issue of the mega-hours of training it would require. Needless to say, I lost that battle. Training began in earnest, and a-marathoning he did go!

Time passed quickly. Before we knew it, our son, Tal, was graduating from high school and beginning his college days. Our daughter, Laura, would be on that track before long, too. Don and I rarely took much time off to attend medical conferences. If there were off-call opportunities, we usually headed close by to the sandy shores of Saint George Island. However, every couple of years we would travel to an American College of OB/GYN meeting, or a meeting of the Georgia OB/GYN Society, or a regional conference for a short-term diversion and some CME (Continuing Medical Education) credits! Don also developed an interest in bone-density issues and became a Certified Clinical Densitometrist, certified by the International Society for Clinical Densitometry. He was then able to lend his skills in interpreting bone-density studies and treating osteoporosis. That also required some time away for education.

Don was really enjoying his running experiences. Fortunately for all of us, in the nine years he had been competing in marathons, he had only suffered the typical injuries of a runner: shin-splints, plantar fasciitis, ankle strains, etc.; nothing that disabled him for significant periods of time. Moreover, these injuries weren't particularly impactful to his doctoring duties, either.

My husband is a very good speaker and has no timidity getting up in front of a group to give a talk or share a story. At this point in my narrative, Don is soon to have his fiftieth birthday and has already run eleven marathons. These, of course, are in addition to the multiple 5Ks and other local events he has done over the years. He developed a real enthusiasm for exercise – his form of choice was running, and he became quite fit.

It was February 2004 and we planned to take a weekend trip to Savannah. Laura was a junior in high school, but she was not going with us. The agenda included a fitness lecture which Don would give at a local hospital on Friday morning. Then, we'd piddle around Savannah a bit and go out for supper at a local seafood restaurant. One of Tal's buddies, Matt, was going to meet up with us, and we'd have supper together. On Saturday morning (early!), Don and Matt would participate together in a half-marathon (13.1 miles), which was being held on Tybee Island. It was expected to take 2 to 2½ hours. The rest of the weekend was designated as time to do whatever we wanted to do in Savannah and then drive home.

Friday's lecture went well, apparently, and we enjoyed a little rest and sightseeing that afternoon; but the weather was looking somewhat ominous. So, we didn't venture too far from our hotel. As supper-hour approached, it was beginning to rain. We had already decided we wanted to eat local seafood, and there was a really quaint restaurant on Tybee Island we thought we'd try. Since that would also provide a dry-run trip to Tybee, over near Saturday's race site, this seemed like a good choice.

We braved the weather, and we made our way to the restaurant. Protected by the umbrella we had in our car, the three of us managed to secure a table without getting more than damp. It was a noticeable rain. After ordering our meals, Don excused himself to go visit the restroom; he did not take the umbrella. That little decision may have made all the difference in the event that subsequently took place.

Matt and I were chatting, just waiting for Don to return and for our food to be served. It was really pouring rain by the time we expected to see Don. The restroom facilities were located, by outdoor trek, in a separate building. There were wooden walks (ramps, really, for wheelchair access) that led to and from the restrooms. Matt and I had no view of that building or the ramps because they were located around the corner from the main restaurant area. It seemed like Don had been gone a good while, but we just figured he was hoping the rain would slack off. Remember, he had no umbrella. And it was a hard rain.

When he finally arrived, he was soaked to the bone! Poor guy. He looked absolutely bewildered. With no towel at our disposal, we probably used as many napkins as possible to help dry him off. Then, he began to relate the incident he had just experienced, and we were peppering him with questions. He told us about slipping, falling, and maybe blacking out for a short time.

More than a little dazed, and definitely shaken up by the hard impact on that wooden walkway, he did his best to describe *and to minimize* the situation. The goose-egg on the back of his head was palpable, yet he insisted he was ok, just rattled. Nothing would persuade him to leave or go get checked out. He was ready for a good seafood meal. So, we stayed. I certainly didn't know any tell-tale symptoms to watch for. He could take an hour to eat; he'd be fine. Right?

After we ate, we went to our respective hotels and called it a night. By bedtime, Don was feeling a little better, but his back was bothering him. He decided he must have pulled a muscle when he fell. Still, he thought a good night's rest would help. No plans would change. It was important to him that he be a good support partner for Matt in the half-marathon the next morning.

Bright and early Saturday morning, we dutifully made our way to Tybee Island for the race. My role as spectator required little preparation; Don and Matt were stoked for the two-hour-plus "pounding of the pavement." No, Don did not feel his absolute best, but his tenacity, commitment, and drive spurred him forward. The weather had greatly improved, and the race route seemed quite acceptable.

The race started and off they go. I had plenty of time to just hang out and make my way to the finish line so I could greet them, providing appropriate praise for their accomplishment. Little did I realize that Don and I had now embarked on a marathon of a different type in our lives.

When he found me, just minutes after the race started, I was taken aback and was very concerned. Apparently, he could not ignore the painful spasms in his lower back and he just didn't feel good. I asked all the usual worried-wife questions, and we went to find a place near the finish line to wait for Matt. Don felt so deflated about having to quit the race; he hated to let Matt down. However, if you try and just *can't* do it, then you just *can't* do it!

Of course, Matt was very understanding, though disappointed. He came through and did very well in his half-marathon. That was a major accomplishment for him, and Don was quite proud of him for his efforts.

Well, we all eventually said our goodbyes, and the rest of the day was open for doing whatever we wanted. So, Saturday afternoon we decided to keep it low-key and just take in the shops along the Savannah Riverwalk. We were browsing and souvenir shopping, taking our time and enjoying our stroll in the crisp February climate. In one of the boutiques, Don found some attractive items he thought I might like. He was deep in thought, repeatedly turning one of the items over and over in his hand, like he was studying it. Such an intense look was on his face. I walked over and asked, "What's wrong?" He looked up and said, "I can't remember your birthdate."

This was the first indication that maybe the lick to his head had affected his memory a little. There would be several other incidents of sketchy memory over the next few days, but this resolved fairly quickly, as I recall. By far, the predominant difficulty was Don's back. It continued to impact his ease of movement. Eventually, because it was not getting better, he decided he needed to see a doctor. So, he called and made the earliest orthopedic appointment he could get.

After returning home from Savannah, Don went back to work as usual and was probably on call the next weekend. He pulled every-other night and every-other weekend in his two-physician practice at that time.

The week after that, he was scheduled to make a trip back toward the Atlantic coast, this time to the town of Brunswick, Georgia.

Despite the lower-back issues, Don reassured me, of course, that he felt fully capable of driving himself to Brunswick. He was complaining about his back more than anything else, and I really don't think he had been completely honest about his other symptoms. It had been less than two weeks since our fateful trip to Tybee Island, and he was being his typical tough-guy self. *Just cinch up your belt and keep going* was his philosophy. I'm not medically trained at all, so I certainly didn't know what to look for. Does experience taking care of scrapes, cuts, flu, chicken pox, and poison ivy qualify me for concussion assessment? Hardly!

When he arrived at his hotel in Brunswick, he called me. The drive across our state had been harrowing for him, and he encountered bizarre road issues. After relating his traumatic trip details to me, my heart dropped into my stomach!! He was five hours away from home, and he was shaken! Moreover, he was already dreading the return trip in a couple of days. I was beside myself!

We stayed on the phone until I felt he had calmed down and was feeling more confident. Eventually, we said our goodbyes and "I love you"s. Immediately, I hit my knees and began pouring out my heart and petitions to my loving Father God. I was profoundly grateful that Don had made it safely. "Thank You, dear sweet Lord, for Your great mercy in letting Don arrive safely," I prayed. I was equally passionate in asking God for that same mercy for a safe trip back to Bainbridge!

Praise the Lord, the return trip was without incident, though I'm sure that in hearing Don's account there would certainly have been challenges. I just remember the extreme sense of relief I had when he pulled into our carport! "Thank You, precious Lord!!"

That, then, was the catalyst for a new policy at home: Mary will do *all* the driving from now on. With the exception of driving himself back and forth to work or to the hospital, and some occasional Rotary Club meetings in our area, I did all the driving for over fourteen years. My husband may have a stubborn I-can-do-it attitude, but, to his credit, he also has a level head on his shoulders. He was *very* aware of road-safety issues. And, as we discovered, the more complex the traffic, the more challenging the visual input, the harder it was for him to function safely.

So, he swallowed his pride, and dutifully took his place in the passenger's seat. He became a wonderful navigator while riding "shotgun." Of course, this made it possible for him to take good naps, too, recouping a little from stressful days in the office and long nights delivering babies.

As for me, I developed more confidence in my out-of-town and out-of-state driving. I proved to be more than capable of negotiating traffic in Atlanta, Columbus, Orlando, and beyond! Even renting a car on vacations and traveling completely unfamiliar terrain was not intimidating like before. So, we adjusted to our circumstances and settled into our new roles.

Now, back to the story. Upon returning from Brunswick, Don made an appointment (as I already mentioned) with an orthopedist because his back was just giving him fits. I truly believe he was in abject denial about the traveling difficulties he had just encountered. I didn't know anything at all about concussions. I never made that connection. Thank the Lord his doctor did! That orthopedic visit started us on a neurological journey, and now the doctor had become the patient. My lack of knowledge in this new realm was a disadvantage. There was much I would learn, though, in short order.

Probably within three to four weeks after the actual fall on that rainy evening, we were both realizing that a gradual onset of other symptoms was occurring. The orthopedist had noted the rapid-eye movement (nystagmus), which forced us to take this whole thing more seriously. We realized, as well, that all had not gotten back to normal. The misperceptions while driving had not abated. Don was no longer the driver, but being a passenger had its challenges, too. He was experiencing headaches and a huge sense of fatigue. Over time, he also had problems with sudden movements, or turning his head quickly, etc. Loud noises became intolerable and he struggled to walk in a straight line.

Probably one of the first really significant truths we learned in our doctors' visits is the fact that concussions or head traumas have a rather cumulative nature. That means that any other bumps or licks to his head that Don had experienced in his life could still have vestiges of impact. That had the potential, no doubt, to make this latest "hit" more pronounced and injurious. Sports people are beginning to get onboard with this fact and are being more cautious about players returning to the field. In my very non-medical way of assessing things, I began to think of Don's brain as being bruised. Bruising of any kind takes time to heal. There are very few truly diagnostic tests to help pinpoint any specific injuries, or even the *areas* of injury, from an impactful fall. During visits with a neurologist, Don simply told the doctor about the symptoms he was experiencing, I shared my own observations and concerns, and then we followed the physician's advice.

Quite a number of physicians and specialists were seen; prescriptions were tried. One step forward, two steps back. Some professionals listened politely as Don described his feelings and difficulties, but you could tell they were not fully grasping the picture or even lending credence to this professional who was baring himself, looking for help, in this uncharted, foreign world. I began to think of this as our wilderness experience.

As a migraine sufferer, I certainly know, understand, and appreciate difficulties with one's head. There is a whole-system impact that those horrible headaches have on you. Pain, sensitivity, nausea, and a need to just be still and quiet are the hallmark symptoms. I've had it all, and it is no fun. For me, these migraine episodes result in a sense of fatigue and profound dullness of thinking. Once the pain and other symptoms resolve, it still takes a day to just get back to feeling normal.

This life-experience really helped me relate to and be very sympathetic of Don's battle each day to try to find "normal" again. We eventually decided he had a "new" normal, because improvement of the issues with his head were not materializing very quickly. This concussion had really been a significant event.

It was a very disconcerting feeling for me. Don was challenged, but there was so little I could do to truly be helpful or make it better. My nurturing side wanted to brew him a special, even magical, cup of hot tea and make him all healthy again. It was the Lord's blessing and His enabling that allowed Don to be able to continue working and taking call and performing his professional duties. He adapted to what he could do, asked for assistance for things he couldn't do, and then rested a lot when he came home. As for me, I honed my sensitivity to his new needs, and I prayed. A lot.

I learned to recognize when he was out of sorts. Evenings and weekends were now times of rest and winding down. Don's usual practice of reading medical articles for a couple of hours before bedtime had to stop. Needless to say, I became, unfortunately, a bit of a nag and control fanatic. I was forever reminding him of how his activities were going to make him feel. When he was resting, I would do my best to be quiet. I even had to be careful not to suddenly laugh really loudly. All stimuli had the potential to be problematic.

It was not my desire to be a schedule dictator, a nag, or a nay-sayer for something he wanted to do, but sometimes I was the voice of reason and prudence. For example, he loves yard work. However, there are certain repetitive motions involved like bending over to pull weeds or scoop up the raked leaves, etc. His back was now completely healed, but his head did not like motion or things that move. He would pay a dear recovery price if he wasn't careful.

Reading medical literature, doing some kind of CME, or trying to write a medical article for the local newspaper was much more difficult at the end of a workday. I constantly told him he was taxing his brain and he needed to just rest. He knew it was true, but he also knew that those tasks were essential to his life and living. It was extremely frustrating for him; I understood that. Still, his health and hope for improvement depended on him being as good to himself as he could be, letting his needs in the moment dictate what he did or didn't do next.

Though I did not feel how Don felt, nor did I fully grasp the things he was experiencing, there was never a time that I did not comprehend that his issues were real. I don't just mean real to *him*. They were *real*. I could see it in his eyes every time he was having a head episode. Obviously, things were misfiring in his brain and making him unsteady on his feet or in his perceptions. It is very hard to explain; and boy, was it ever hard for him to explain it to anybody else!

One example of strange phenomena happened as we would be traveling in the car. If I was driving and had to brake quickly because of traffic, Don would immediately belch. I mean, within a millisecond, his head-to-stomach signal would trigger a belch or a series of belches. That was a physical manifestation and a rapid-fire response to a change in motion: a deceleration. That was *real* and involuntary.

Another example took place at night while sleeping. Though we were never really sure what caused it, there were many nights when Don would jerk suddenly and scare the stew out of me. In addition, he had a frequent tendency to kick his legs, usually striking me unexpectedly on my shins. There were a number of times, I well remember, that I was almost pushed out of bed! And guess what? These occurrences made me wide-awake for a long time, and he just kept right on sleeping!! It never woke him up. Go figure! And hey, that was real.

When I observed the tell-tale look in his eyes, I knew he was struggling. The specifics of what was happening behind his eyes were veiled from me, but it only mattered that he was having an episode. My usual response was to give him a hug of reassurance that we were in this wilderness together. Somehow there was a great purpose in all this, and God would use it for good and for His glory. Of that, I was absolutely confident.

One of Don's great loves is being near the ocean. The serenity, the beauty, the magnitude of God's creation, the sea life, the sun, and the awe-inspiring power of the ocean have fascinated and drawn him since he was a youngster. We discovered St. George Island, Florida, pretty soon after moving to Bainbridge, and we both fell in love with all the island had to offer.

Unfortunately, after his concussion in 2004, walks on the beach were a source of too much visual input. It became obvious that even this beloved activity was now to be enjoyed on a very limited basis. Don was devastated by this realization, but there was no way to just ignore the "spinning" and take a walk anyway. Any short walks he dared to attempt had to involve both of us. He would need the stability of my arm locked in his. The wave activity and peripheral input would overwhelm him, and his head would struggle to process and cope with the stimuli. Despite our reluctance to do so, it was becoming increasingly certain that we must accept and embrace the "new" normal, and the necessary restrictions, that defined our days.

As the days turned into weeks and the weeks turned into months, we found ourselves resigned to being careful about trigger foods, about not missing any medicine doses, about not overdoing to the point of really being exhausted, and about avoiding the troublesome motion stimuli. I say "we" because I was like a pesky insect always reminding, warning, or chiding Don about something! Our daily lives were impacted in practically every way, and we knew it. The one area that was not altered was our faith life and dependence on the Lord. Because of this, I was never burdened about what the future held. With great assurance within my spirit, I knew that whatever the future held, God was in control and we would sail those seas with Him as our Captain. There was no way to predict how this season would play out or how long we would be traveling this road.

Don's eyes, his demeanor, his memory gaps, and his tendency to withdraw were all signals I learned to recognize. If possible, I would try to help compensate, or I would avoid making it worse. My primary function at those times was to be understanding, making Don feel like I had his back, even if I couldn't do one single thing to make any of it go away. My pet phrase for a while was, "Looks like your gyroscope is cutting up again."

Just because I couldn't personally experience or relate to what was going on with him, doesn't mean I was unable to be a big help. I pray that I was, and have constantly been, just that. For example, when his "gyroscope" was misbehaving, I would become his human crutch. That was a game-changer. The simple act of locking arms, so that I provided a bolstering sense of balance, gave him a profound feeling of security. All the while, I was praying for God to heal him, and for us to learn the intended life lessons through this season.

Without a doubt, I was on the outside looking in, doing my very best to comprehend all my husband was feeling and experiencing. Perhaps my newfound role in our situation is not terribly different from a male physician becoming an OB/GYN. He'll never have periods or cramps, he'll never experience pregnancy and childbirth, and he'll never deal with any female-related issues (like PMS). However, that male physician can be trained by textbook and real-life, day-to-day patient care to be an excellent professional provider who truly understands even the things he will never personally feel.

I was in OJT (on-the-job training), learning how to assess and support this man who was dealing with the effects of a mild TBI. At times, it was difficult to tell if I was being his wife or his mother. I know I have definitely worn both pairs of shoes, so to speak. In this wilderness journey, both of us have learned a great deal. At the very core of our responses was a deep sense of humility and trust. God was in control, and He had a purpose for our situation. We braced our spirits with an unyielding faith in His plans, and we accepted this new lot in life. We became more patient with each other and with handling our unwelcomed circumstances. Our deep-seated love for and commitment to each other strengthened, bolstering our relationship's foundation.

In any battle or difficult situation you face, there are two basic choices: accept the hand you are dealt and, by God's grace, move forward to victory; or, succumb to the challenges and bear a sense of defeat. A very relevant scripture is I Peter 5:6-7. Those two verses say, "Humble yourselves, therefore, under the mighty hand of God, that He may exalt you at the proper time, casting all your anxiety upon Him, because He cares for you." (NASB) Because God does indeed care for us, we must humble ourselves under His mighty hand and seek to know what He wants to show us through our trials.

I would like to go on record at this point and praise the character of my wonderful husband. He is such a Godly man and I am so very proud of the way he has handled every phase of this journey. There have been a number of ups and downs, with more challenges than answers, but through it all he has never been tempted to find relief in alcohol or pills or illicit drugs. Considering the emotional turmoil and times of despondence, I could certainly see how he, or anyone struggling with such difficulties, might seek refuge from daily life by turning to a chemical escape. How thankful I am that we did not have to also fight those demons!

Moreover, Don has also continually tapped into his tenacious spirit and absolutely would not give up, give in, sit down, or join a pity-party. Many days he did not feel good at all, but he kept going. He might feel a little low, but he kept going. There were occasional times of sheer weariness, but he refused to let himself feel defeated. Yes, he learned some smart ways to handle his symptoms, accepting the need for restrictions and protracted periods of recuperative rest, because his sense of well-being demanded it. The struggle was daunting at times, but he remained undaunted. That's his character. I am beyond blessed and grateful that God gifted me with such a man of character, to love and to cherish, for better or for worse.

Over the course of these years, efforts to find healing have run the gamut. We have tried prescription medicines, lifestyle adjustments, dietary changes, therapeutic exercise regimens, and even good, old-fashioned common sense. The year 2020 is already in full swing. Praise the Lord, my husband is now at a place of good health. It took a long time, but over the last eighteen months there has been an increasing awareness that symptoms have greatly improved or completely resolved!! We are claiming a miraculous healing from Almighty God, and I am so thankful for it. Don realizes that not everyone with a TBI, whether mild or severe, will encounter full recovery. But re-gaining part or most of what was perceived as lost gives a sufferer countless reasons to celebrate.

As a concerned outsider looking in, I certainly could not accurately discern when symptoms were truly abating and improving, and when they were just being effectively masked. Don is not a whiner by nature, and my questions regarding how he was feeling on any given day were often answered with, "Pretty good," or "I'm okay," or, sometimes, "Mary, stop asking me how I'm doing!" Those were very off-putting responses and were not very informative. The underlying truth, however, is that even if I had known exactly how he was feeling or what struggles were on his plate that day, I was poor help to make any beneficial difference. That being said, it is equally true that my knowing what was going on for him would certainly affect my behavior around him so as to not make him feel worse. I firmly believe that a caring attitude goes hand-in-hand with being fully informed about circumstances.

The passage of time, and staying the course with medications and activity restrictions, did bring about gradual improvement. The tell-tale signs of a malfunctioning gyroscope, the evidence of headaches, the tendency for extreme fatigue, and the difficulties instigated by quick head-movements, became less pronounced, as I observed. Like I said before, this could have been because these symptoms were actually lessening or because my husband was adapting to, adjusting in, compensating for, and tolerating his issues better. Either way, he was learning to live with his newfound situation, and there was a huge degree of healing just in that fact alone.

The old expression, "a watched pot never boils," resonates with me as I apply this adage to our circumstances. If you fixate on what's wrong and you let yourself become burdened by what you can't do, then life becomes micro-focused and the progression from "low boiling" to "full boiling," or adaptation, is greatly delayed. If, however, you embrace the changes you've experienced and stay busy doing what you *can* do, pretty soon your pot is reaching a "rolling boil." There is a big difference between accepting or embracing changes vs. feeling defeated by those changes. Attitude through the difficult times can be a game-changer. Asking the Lord to show you what you're supposed to learn in any given situation is so very important. Trusting Him, leaning on Him, and seeking His wisdom is the threefold key to moving forward in a positive way.

I could have shared multiple stories with you, ones that reinforced the difficulties in this saga, but that would have only been an excess. What you have read is not overstated or dramatized. It is a real and honest account of my side of the story. Don and I are stronger because we went through this together. Our faith is deeper because we, in our extreme vulnerability, relied completely on God and His divine mercy and grace.

If you are in a wilderness journey of your own, please let me encourage you to never give up. There is hope, and whatever strange symptoms or issues you might be having, rest assured that there are many others, just like us, who have walked in those shoes. Physicians do care, and there is so much more they are learning about concussions and TBIs. Do your best to describe and explain your feelings and your problems. Settle within yourself that your challenges are real. What you are dealing with is *real*! Seek the peace of God and pray for recovery. He knows the path you are on. And He is listening. Isaiah 43:1-3 says, "Do not fear for I have redeemed you. I have called you by name, you are Mine! When you pass through the waters, I will be with you; and through the rivers, they will not overflow you. When you walk through the fire, you will not be scorched, nor will the flame burn you. For I am the Lord your God, the Holy One of Israel, your Savior." (NASB) That says it all.

Mary, thank you for your insights and sharing. Thank you for your dedication, love, and devotion.

CHAPTER 16

Yesterdays

"Memories are the trail markers that determine the path of your future." Author

As I reflect on the struggles that make up my yesterdays, I realize that I never kept a record of my healing levels. It would be so nice here to give you a timeline of improvement, but I just don't have one. That was partly by intention. As I said earlier, I was determined not to become a professional patient. While I sought the help I needed so I could continue to function, I tried to never visualize myself primarily as a patient with a disability in need of on-going management. That management was necessary, but it was never my focus. My injury, my treatment, and my behaviors to compensate were just part of my daily routine. I took my medicine and I went to my appointments, but those efforts were just a part of the flow of my life. I also took vitamins, ran in the early years, got up for work, shaved and showered, etc. In short, I tended to the necessities of life, and some of those necessities involved management of my condition. I guess you could compare my accommodations to my new life to what it is like to set off on an outing in a new pair of shoes. While roaming about, you may discover those shoes just don't fit right and are uncomfortable. You may find yourself regretting your choice. You may even say to yourself, "I am going to have a blister from this." Once committed, however, you cannot just discard those shoes halfway through your outing. Like them or not, adjust to them or not, you must keep going, and they will be with you for the entirety of the outing.

So, applying this analogy to my life, as time passed, and recovery steps occurred, I still had needs. Though accommodations during my outings changed, there were *still* accommodations. Even today, I live within some constraints to minimize the challenges I must overcome.

Different obstacles along the way of my recovery required different strategies, but they all required adjustments and patience. After my fall, my time of profound impact evolved over that first three to four weeks and really lasted for years. My medical care helped me to "control" some of my symptoms, especially as time went by. I remember that my greatest susceptibility to motion dysfunction lasted through the first several years. Even with medical help and therapy, my lack of filter led to sensations of "spinning" and feeling "spacey" on a daily basis. I had to be consciously aware and on my guard in order to limit my dysfunction. Even now, yet to a much lesser degree, that is an issue.

My awareness of memory loss was my first noted deficit and probably the first issue to resolve. I had pinpoint memory deficits at the beginning. My issue was never pervasive or profound. I did not continue to have difficulty recalling birthdates and similar items. I don't think there were any further episodes that mimicked my being frozen by an inability to remember a significant event like my wife's birthday. On a current and daily basis, my practice of keeping (and using) a peripheral memory aid in my pocket really brought me back close to my baseline functionality.

"Word search" has been persistent through my journey and remains a challenge. My words just will not flow easily at times. Even in relaxed conversation with Mary, there are many pauses. Some days are worse than others. That fault in the flow of words can be embarrassing and cause episodes of social avoidance. However, in my analysis, there are two areas where my words do *not* fail me. In fact, these are the two areas where I have been *called* to service: medicine and Biblical teaching. That is a miracle in and of itself; one that should not be overlooked! Thanks be to God!

The headaches were not a major issue for me. They were a distraction. At times, they were more than that. Fortunately, they were controlled with rest, acetaminophen, and the use of other preventative medicines. My recollection is that the headache issues resolved to a great degree within the first year.

As you no doubt realize, especially if you are a victim or caretaker, my progression to wholeness would not fit on a two-dimensional linear graph. There was no steadily-advancing climb of improvement. I see my recovery like the image I have chosen for the cover of this book. I visualize a hiker on a steep slope. Along such climbs, one encounters all kinds of obstacles. There are notable boulders that require planning and preparation in order to conquer them. There may be overhangs that appear all but insurmountable. There can be rocks that appear stable, but crumble with your weight. And there is always gravel that can roll under your feet, causing you to slip and lose ground. Sometimes you are on your feet, but other times you must climb on hands and knees in order to gain ground. Overall, the climber continues to progress, but it is not a linear trail. There are gains and slips: new highs and then backslides. That analogy is so much like my healing journey.

Over time, as we learn and adapt, there is a natural trend in our human activities: we assume the future will be like the present. I had to learn, though, that just because I was having a good week with symptom control, did not mean I was bullet-proof on a Saturday. Pushing the issue, when I actually needed rest, was a real slide on that gravel. If I ignored any attempts to prevent those stimuli that provoked me, I could lose what control I had experienced. I would just be forced to stop to recover. The payment for being bull-headed was that intense sensation I called "pressure." This was really true for several years after the injury. My Saturdays had to be days of recovery. That lasted for over five years. I suspect my personal requirement for recovery was directly related to how much I demanded from my brain during the week.

On the long end of things, in terms of recovery, was my ability to drive in traffic. Depending on the level of traffic, the number of lanes, the number of cars that surround you, and the complexity of freeway interchanges, driving is a multi-focus encounter, requiring concentration and intensity. It took me over fourteen years to feel up to the challenge of freeway driving. Almost like a young driver, I had to retrain myself at that point by gradually increasing the complexity of the situations I exposed myself to. Today, while I don't like driving in heavy traffic, I am able to safely handle it.

So, you see, recovery is in stages. Healing will not be accomplished in a day or all at one time. But healing *can* occur. My journey involved growth and maturity over a span of years. I hope your recovery is quicker and more complete. However the trek though, remember it is about the day-to-day journey. Value each day and the lessons you learn. Be thankful for those who help you hold up to the challenge with their support and encouragement. God puts His saints in our paths because He knows our needs. If we look closely, we can see the image of God in the eyes of those who love us in His name. God will provide!

I am sure you have heard the old saying, "I gave at the office." Actually, and unfortunately for my family, I gave it all at the office and hospital. By the time I arrived home, I was done! I had to view that circumstance from a positive light. God gave me the opportunity to be a doctor, and God guided me to Bainbridge. My only explanation for how I continued to function at the high level of being a specialist and a surgeon, was (and is) His grace. He called me, and He tooled me. He placed me, empowered me, and delivered me. Indeed, I was very careful to be safe. I took a whole year requesting that my partner always attend cases in the operating room when I was there. We worked together as we always had, but he never had to step in for me. God's grace! Paul tells us of his experience in the palm of the Father's hand in 2 Corinthians 12:9 "My grace is sufficient for you, for my power is made perfect in weakness."

CHAPTER 17

Today

"Maybe the journey isn't so much about becoming anything. Maybe it's about un-becoming everything that isn't really you, so you can be who you were meant to be in the first place." Paul Coelho

As I reflect on my healing progression and how Mary has helped me these many years, I return to the present. For a while now, I thought all my symptoms had resolved. I had even progressed to being able to take long walks and bike rides on the beach. I have now become bold in challenging my former limits. Not all challenges result in victorious outcomes, though. I was wrong in assuming my symptoms were totally resolved. I misread being under control, for being totally normal. Both are good and desirable goals, but they are definitely different in scope from each other. The symptoms were only gone like a summer rash that clears in winter, only to reappear with the heat. I thought I was *totally* resolved, but I wasn't!

I have not had much in the way of imbalance or spatial disorientation symptoms in the last year and a half. First, I weaned off pregabalin SLOWLY. I did ok and never noted a resurgence of symptoms. I continued the escitalopram for about six months as my only head-issue medicine. Then I felt it was time to begin to wean down on that. (This was all approved by my doctor; *don't* exclude that expert professional from your planning!) I was already at 10 milligrams per day, down from 20 mg earlier on. I cut it to 5 mg. Now that I am retired, and since my symptoms have significantly resolved, I thought, "Why not?" So, I was down to 5 milligrams per day, and had been on this dose for a few weeks. The next step was to split those in half and take 2.5 milligrams a day for a while. Then, maybe I could space them out before totally stopping this medicine. That weaning, using a staggered, decreasing dose, has worked fairly well for my patients when I used it in my practice. I have done this routine with many medicines in this class. Weaning usually avoids rebound symptoms. I used to tell patients, "If you get off of this slowly and you begin noticing more symptoms, it is because you still need the medicine." That is different from a cold-turkey stop that can lead to rebound with your original symptoms blowing back, compounded by new problems, as well. Stopping cold-turkey, for most drugs in this class, is *not* a good idea.

When I have weaned patients off escitalopram, I was treating them for depression and/or anxiety. Depression and anxiety are two conditions that may come into someone's life for a time and then resolve. These conditions also may be life-long issues. I often used the analogy that sometimes your car gets in a rut and you need help getting back onto the normal road of life. If depression or anxiety is causing relational problems or work issues, it is time for treatment of one kind or another. Medicine can be very helpful, as can reducing stimulants (like caffeine and simple sugars), increasing exercise, and developing good sleep-hygiene. Once someone's symptoms are under control, I like to think about a re-training period of at least six months, whereby the person can coast, feeling better about issues and about themselves. Getting off the medicine at that point and maintaining other healthy behaviors can be successful for the long-term.

However, scientists tell us that it is the level of serotonin in certain parts of our brain that can provoke feelings of depression. While some of us have short-term, situational issues, others of us have inherited abnormal serotonin function. This latter group may require life-long medication to maintain a healthy emotional life. It's important to realize however, that serotonin production can also be permanently altered in those who have experienced mild head trauma. This permanent change in the production of this neurotransmitter can alter many functions in your brain. This group of traumatized individuals may also benefit from the long term us of drugs such as the selective serotonin reuptake inhibitors (SSRI). Drugs in this class are usually prescribed in the general population as anti-depressants.

Well, that is my speech on weaning, as it relates to medicine for depression and anxiety. Sure, we all get sad and discouraged at times. Trying to overcome a slowly healing brain can certainly contribute to feelings of loss, discouragement, and frustration. Sometimes a part of that response is true depression, but not always. In my case, my challenge was more a problem of anxiety. I would get jittery, anxious, and worried. Particularly if I was dealing with a patient who had serious issues or difficulties from surgery, I struggled to not be consumed. If you have dealt with anxiety, you know it is a self-questioning-and-doubting type of challenge. For a professional, it is embarrassing and can erode confidence. Escitalopram did help me overcome this. Apparently, it also helped control my imbalance symptoms. Theoretically, that can make sense. Balance confusion involves your brain receiving data from sensory organs and, then, having difficulty fine-tuning a response. Neurotransmitters are definitely involved in this process, and abnormal levels of these compounds can alter the communication in the brain. Medicines like escitalopram may help to normalize levels of these neurotransmitters.

Back to my attempts to wean off the escitalopram. I had noticed, since I had been on the 5-mg dose, that I had more "mini-episodes" of spinning and spacey issues. Also, I had noticed that bending over and standing up had started to cause me to feel a little out-of-sync for a minute or so. That was a bad memory returning. Those symptoms brought on by bending and then standing up can complicate a lot of things I try to do outside. Since my earlier, more symptomatic days were now in the past, I had liberalized such movements and activities. But wait, they had come back! As usual, I tried to ignore and move past these symptoms without taking them seriously. I wasn't ready to accept that this level of dysfunction was returning, could be permanent, and might require on-going medical treatment.

That attitude was working until last week. I went a couple of days without adequate sleep. Then one day, I did a lot of driving. Between driving around town and then driving six hours on a short trip, I began to notice my head was feeling uncomfortable with all the movement. For over a year, I had been doing well driving such distances. Not this time. Next, my allergies acted up and I went from occasional sneezing to a barn-blowout sneeze. Oh, it brought back an all-too-familiar spinning response and the painful memories of experiences of the past! I sneezed; and then I froze, just holding onto the counter. It took a couple of minutes to feel in control from the disorientating spinning. I am now two days out from that event, and I hope that the feeling of spatial instability is about gone!

As I write this section, I am in Florida during the COVID-19 pandemic. It is spring, my favorite time of year to go to the beach. The county where I am staying just opened the beaches last week, after two months or so of forbidding beach walks and recreation. I had planned to walk out to the beach when we got here. I wanted to smell that salt air and feel the ocean breeze, while I soaked my ankles in the surf. I wanted to sit on the beach and read. That is what I wanted and planned. So far, because of the way my head feels, I have not been bold enough to take the beach on. I am hoping that my current symptoms will continue to resolve, and I will be ready to go tomorrow! I think the symptoms have returned because of several factors. One of those is my recent compromise of sleep time. On top of that are: the increased motion of the driving, along with the shock of sneezing. Liberalizing my activities and my diet over time have taken me closer to the edge of my tolerance and are certainly co-contributors. The final factor, I believe, must be the reduced dose of escitalopram.

My plan now is to increase my escitalopram dose, watch the potential triggers in my diet more carefully, and concentrate on good sleep habits or hygiene, as the experts refer to it. I will also be a little more conservative in my physical activities.

Yes, I am discouraged to have to stop weaning and go back up on the medicine. However, my being functionally capable trumps all the dysfunctional options that I have experienced. And the good news is, I am confident that the symptoms will get better with the right interventions! I know "better" now! I have learned the path.

My journey is on-going! My climb continues! I am so much closer, but I have not, as of yet, reached the summit of healing! By God's power, that will occur!

As I scan the years since 2004, I know a truth. For me and mine the phrase, "We lived happily ever after," has come to pass. I have love and joy. I have caring, faithfulness, and hope. I look forward to that "ever after" continuing!

CHAPTER 18

Conclusion

"Change is the only constant in life." Heraclitus

According to Alhilali, et al, as published in 2014, traumatic brain injury, often mild, annually affects between 1.8 and 3.8 million individuals in the USA. That means, there are a bunch of us! For many of us, the symptoms resolve in hours or in a few days. That was my response with the first two concussions. Unfortunately, as no doubt you realize, that resolution does not occur quickly or easily in all victims. If you have read to this point, I suspect that you are either such a victim as myself, or you are a supporter of one. If I have fulfilled my purpose in writing this book, there may have been areas where you could see yourself in the mirror of my descriptions. I bet that you have seen some of your experiences or symptoms in my revelation.

I say, "Take heart; you are far from alone." The symptoms I was experiencing, no doubt, are common to many, and yet they felt uniquely bizarre to me. As I searched for answers, I did not realize how many others were suffering in the same ways. The impetus for writing this book is because of that loneliness and desertion I felt. My aim has been to shine the light so that others may benefit from learning of our commonality. I also hope that others, earlier on the road, may benefit from what I have grown to learn through my travels to healing. By the way, *hope* can be a noun or a verb. I have chosen to rely on hope as a verb. I took whatever steps were required to pursue healing and improvement. You must also consider your options and go for any glimmer of light that will brighten your path.

What about you? Where are you on your journey? How long have you been dealing with your challenge? Did you see yourself or your loved one in these pages? I hope that you have found some measure of optimism! I hope that while I may not have helped make your therapeutic direction any simpler, I have encouraged you to be patient, and yet continue to fight. There are just times when we must back off, reassess, and reclaim our priorities. Life is about more than how high you can climb on the mountain. Life is also about who helps you and whom you can help, along the climb. I have learned the importance of patience, love, and support. I have allotted more time for listening to the ones I love and made a conscious decision to be less time-demanding. I have learned, more than ever, the place of the Trinity in my life: God the Father, God the Son, and God the Holy Spirit. I have learned of His love through so many caring people.

I still have a medical license. And I still write prescriptions. You may not be my patient, but you are my brother or sister. I can write you a prescription. My prescription for you is **hope**. Not hope in the worldly or the failings of our surrounds. No, this hope is in the Father of the universe. May you be guided, assured, and given peace through your walk with Him!

"Do not be anxious about anything, but in everything, by prayer and petition, with thanksgiving, present your requests to God. And the peace of God, which transcends all understanding, will guard your hearts and your minds in Christ Jesus." Philippians 4:6-7.

I walked along the path on St. George Island this morning. I noticed how nice the houses are, how brightly they are colored, how neatly they are configured, and how precise the man-made outlines can be. All of that is due to proper planning and follow-through. That is what my life was like, as *I* built *my* future.

But you know what really got my attention this morning? It was not all that precise work of man. What I saw was a weed growing away from other plants. No one would buy it in a store. No one would purposely plant it in a flower bed. Hardly anyone would even notice it. Yet, it was so beautiful! The green stalks that supported the small white flowers arose out of a bed of leaves that were shining a translucent red; very bright in the morning light. My life is now more like that weed. I am at a point that was not planned this way by me. I accept that it has been planned by a greater hand! That greater hand can take the ordinary and the discarded and create the new and the beautiful. May you be blessed with a beautiful life as you grow into what He has planned for you.

"Therefore, since we are surrounded by such a great cloud of witnesses, let us throw off everything that hinders and the sin that so easily entangles, and let us run with perseverance the race marked out for us. Let us fix our eyes on Jesus, the Author and Perfecter of our faith, who for the joy set before Him endured the cross, scorning its shame, and sat down at the right hand of the throne of God. Consider Him who endured such opposition from sinful men, so that you will not grow weary and lose heart." Hebrews 12:1-3

Daughter Laura's concept of my journey

EPILOGUE

I have spent my work life as a physician. What a privilege that has been! I have shared great joys. Countless births are responsible for many of those moments of joy. Watching those children and those families mature and thrive in this small town has been wonderful and fulfilling. The scope of a physician's profession, particularly as an obstetrician and gynecologist, means that there will also be encounters of great sadness. Sharing such pain has also been a bonding and growing experience during my career. I have been blessed to be allowed into areas that my patients were unwilling to share with any others. That vision, to the soul within, has revealed great and convoluted pain at times. I had no tools or therapies that could heal some of those pains. There was no medicine or surgery that might heal the wounds that some of my patients had carried for years. All I could do was care! For some patients, that is exactly what they were looking for: someone who cared and was willing to try and understand. I opened my heart. Sharing a patient's pain was one of the heaviest burdens I ever had to bear. At times, I literally felt the weight of the pain being endured by my patients.

I talked with my neighbor-lady today. She is in her eighties now. We have known each other for over thirty-three years. In fact, she not only lived next door, she also worked in my office. At the time of my injury, she served as our office manager. About two months ago now, she was in a car accident. She got bruises from the seat belt but no broken bones or internal injuries. However, she blacked out, perhaps due to the slap of the air bags. She can't remember the accident. After that day, she began to have short episodes of disorientation. Today, she asked me, "Do you still see things to the periphery that aren't there?" I felt tears in my eyes, realizing the familiarity of what she was experiencing. And I sensed her yearning for reassurance. My heart hurts for her and for all the others that are dealing with the confusion and questioning that comes as a residual of concussion and mild traumatic brain injury.

Doctors and others often take head injuries less than seriously. How many Western movies did I watch as a kid where men were pistol-whipped and knocked out? Our heroes might have had a sore knot, but they never had any long-term issues. They got up and continued the fight. That was fantasy, but I didn't realize it.

As a child, I remember if you got "dazed" playing sports and didn't continue to play, you just weren't "tough enough." Fortunately, much of this is changing. There are now protocols to protect our young athletes.

We need to go beyond looking after our children in sports; we need to look after each other. In our everyday walks of life, we need to be willing to protect each other. We need to open our eyes and always think about the possibility of a head injury. A broken bone shows up on x-ray and can be put in a cast. Not so for mild traumatic brain injury. As physicians and friends, whether we see a bruise or a cut or not, we must remember to ask: "Did you have any kind of hit to your head?" "Do you have a headache?" "Do you feel dizzy?" It might have been a fall, a bike accident, a slip on the floor, a car accident, a hit on a counter as you bend over, running into the door jam in the dark, or any other of a number of possibilities. Care enough to ask, and care enough to step forward and help. If you get a chance, don't forget to look into that person's eyes. Then remember to check again in a few days.

If there is doubt, rest it out!

I am so glad I wrote this book. I know that there are so many out there adrift in uncertainty. I hear those questions echoing. Did you ever feel …? Did you ever see…? Did you ever forget….? Did you ever lose your …? Did you ever experience…? I hope I have helped to offer reassurance by being open and honest about what I experienced and yet was blessed to overcome. And yes, I am glad for my fifteen-year journey, because it has given me a new calling and a new understanding. Maybe together, we can be a healing balm for others! Thanks for being along with me!

ABOUT THE AUTHOR

DON R. ROBINSON, MD, FACOG, CCD

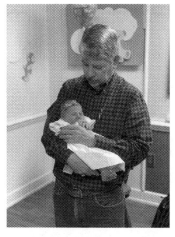

Dr. Don Robinson retired from full-time medical practice in January 2019. He now works in a part-time capacity while he enjoys his family and seeks out new challenges in his life.

He was born in Newnan, Georgia, and was raised in Macon, Georgia. He proudly attended Mercer University and graduated Magna Cum Laude with a bachelor's degree in 1976. He went on to attend the Medical College of Georgia and graduated in 1980. From there, he and Mary returned to Macon to complete his specialty residency in Obstetrics and Gynecology. Upon completion of that step, he, Mary, and young son Tal headed to the wilds of South Dakota with the Air Force. He completed his obligation at Moody AFB in Valdosta, Georgia. From there his family, now with the addition of his daughter Laura, settled down into small-town life in Bainbridge, Georgia.

The richness of small-town life, and the opportunity of spiritual growth through adversity, flower his story!

James 1:2-4 "Count it all joy, my brothers, when you meet trials of various kinds, for you know that the testing of your faith produces steadfastness. And let steadfastness have its full effect, that you may be perfect and complete, lacking in nothing."

GLOSSARY

Cognitive function- generally accepted as the executive mental processes of thinking, reasoning, memory, judgement, and decision making.

Concussion- traumatic brain injury that affects brain function. May be caused by falls, contact injury, or violent shake. May cause loss of consciousness, headaches, problems with concentration, memory, or balance and coordination.

Mild Traumatic Brain Injury, mTBI- a nondegenerative, noncongenital insult to the brain from an external mechanical force, possibly leading to permanent or temporary impairment of cognitive, physical, and psychosocial functions, with an associated diminished or altered state of consciousness.

Motion sickness- probably due to a mix-match from visual and balance input. May be associated with any type of travel but is most noted in "sea sickness." Can be associated with a queasy feeling or nausea. May also be associated with headache, dizziness, or lightheadedness.

Post-concussion syndrome- definition not universally agreed upon. Refers to persistence of some or all of initial concussion symptoms after the usual period of resolution. Some see this as being a few weeks, others as failing to resolve after three months.

Vertigo- the sensation of spinning. Usually this term refers to the sufferer being still and the room spinning. It may also be used to describe "internal" spinning.

Vestibular apparatus- the inner ear. Primarily involves the inner ear cilia, crystals, and semi-circular canals. Charged with maintaining balance throughout our physical actions.

Vestibular Migraine- marked by episodic physical imbalance, with or without headache. May be associated with true vertigo, nausea, imbalance, and poor coordination.

RESOURCES

www.ahn.org	Concussion Center of Allegheny Health Network
www.chrisannegordonmd.com	Specialist in Physical Medicine and Rehabilitation, Author of "Turn the Lights On", personal history of mild traumatic brain injury.
	Founder: Operation Resurrection Foundation. Dedicated to aiding returning warriors with traumatic brain injury
www.daniellevanalst.com	Psychologist author and blogger
www.dizzy.com	American Institute of Balance
www.health.clevelandclinic.org	Family Medicine Nov 12, 2018
	BPPV. Why loose ear crystals make you dizzy and how to fix them
www.hopkinsmedicine.org	Home Epley Maneuver
	Vestibular Migraines
www.legion.org	American Legion articles and helps
	TBI- Veteran's healthcare/tbi
	Signature Wound of the War-traumatic-wound-war-signature-wound-war
	DOD Programs-documents/legion/pdf/TBI.PTSD_hinds.pdf
www.michiganear.com	Balance, Dizziness, and Vertigo
www.neurogrow.com	Brain Fitness Center- info on concussion recovery program
www.neuropt.org/docs/vsig-english-pt-fact-sheets/migraine-diet-triggers.pdg	Info and food triggers for migraine associated dizziness
www.vestibular.org	Balance disorders information

Article: Vestibular disorders following different types of head and neck trauma, Kolev and Sergeeva, Functional Neurology 2016; 31(2):75-80

Book: Vertigo: Its Multisensory Syndromes. Author Brandt. London. Springer. 1999

Book: "Over My HEAD, A Doctor's Own Story of Head Injury from the Inside Looking out" by Claudia L Osborn 1998 Andrews McMeel Publishing

Printed in the United States
By Bookmasters